CHAIR YOGA FOR SENIORS OVER 60

YOUR SIMPLE 10-MINUTE DAILY GUIDE TO IMPROVE
MOBILITY, RELIEVE CHRONIC PAIN, AND LOSE WEIGHT!
REGAIN YOUR INDEPENDENCE BY FOLLOWING
THE ILLUSTRATED, STEP-BY-STEP POSES!

CHARLOTTE STERLING

TABLE OF CONTENTS

e are going to introduce you to the wonderful world of chair yoga! Whether you're an experienced yogi or a complete beginner, chair yoga offers a gentle and accessible way to embrace the benefits of yoga while seated comfortably on a chair.

And this is a complete guidebook about chair yoga for weight loss. Here you will also find, in practice, a 4-week challenge to lose belly fat, improve mobility and maintain independence with simple 10-minute daily sessions.

Our aim is therefore not only to make you feel better on a psycho-physical level but also to help you find an ideal physical shape that is, above all, good for your self-esteem! In this book, various topics will be covered regarding chair yoga: when it was born, how it works and what its benefits are. We will also talk about how to approach the previously named challenge and what the best chair yoga exercises are. Simply put, we will address both theory and practice. But let's start by introducing this specific and fascinating topic.

Chair yoga is a soft form of yoga that is suitable to be performed while seated on a chair or using a chair for support. It was created to make yoga accessible to people who may find it hard to practicing traditional yoga poses due to physical limitations, age, injury, or other health conditions. Chair yoga typically involves performing a series of modified yoga poses, breathing exercises, and relaxation techniques while sitting on a chair or using a chair for stability.

The practice of chair yoga focuses on improving flexibility, strength, balance, and relaxation while also promoting mindfulness and stress reduction. It can be beneficial for people with mobility issues, seniors, office workers who spend extended periods sitting, and those in rehabilitation or recovery from injuries.

Chair yoga classes are often led by instructors with expertise in adapting yoga poses to accommodate various needs and abilities. The practice can be customized to suit individual requirements, making it a versatile and inclusive form of yoga that can be enjoyed by a wide range of people.

In other words, chair yoga is a modified form of traditional yoga that brings all the goodness of a regular yoga practice while catering to diverse needs and abilities. It is perfect for individuals who may have difficulty standing or getting down on a mat, such as seniors, people with limited mobility, injuries, or physical challenges.

In chair yoga, you'll explore a series of yoga postures, breathing exercises, and relaxation techniques that are specifically adapted to be performed while sitting on a chair or using it for support. The practice encourages gentle movements, stretches, and mindful breathing to improve flexibility, strength, balance, and mental focus.

One of the best features of chair yoga is its versatility. Whether you're at home, in the office, or at a community center, all you need is a chair to get started. The practice can be easily tailored to your specific needs, making it adaptable for a wide range of individuals and ages.

During a typical chair yoga session, you'll be guided by a skilled instructor who will lead you through a series of seated poses, modified standing postures using the chair as support, and sometimes even gentle standing poses for those who can manage them. The focus is always on safety and comfort, ensuring that you enjoy the practice without any strain or discomfort.

Beyond the physical benefits, chair yoga also promotes relaxation and stress reduction, helping to soothe your mind and uplift your spirits. By incorporating mindful breathing and meditation techniques, chair yoga fosters a sense of calm and inner peace.

While chair yoga is a wonderful and accessible form of exercise that can offer numerous physical and mental benefits, it's important to have realistic expectations when it comes to using it as a primary method for weight loss. Chair yoga may not be the most effective approach for weight loss compared to other forms of physical activity, such as cardio exercises, strength training, or high-intensity workouts.

That said, chair yoga can still be a valuable component of an overall weight-loss or fitness program. Here's why you might consider reading this book about chair yoga for weight loss:

✓ Low-Impact Exercise: Chair yoga is gentle on the joints and suitable for people with mobility issues or those who are just beginning their fitness journey. It provides a manner to engage in physical activity without putting excessive strain on the body, making it an excellent option for individuals who have weight-related concerns.
✓ Increased Mobility and Flexibility: Consistent practice of chair yoga can improve flexibility and mobility, making it simpler to engage in other physical activities. This can lay the foundation for incorporating more dynamic exercises into your routine.
✓ Stress Reduction: Stress and emotional eating can often lead to weight gain. Chair yoga incorporates relaxation techniques and mindfulness practices that can help manage stress and promote a healthier relationship with food.
✓ Mindful Eating: Chair yoga encourages mindfulness, which can be applied to eating habits as well. By becoming more aware of how and what you eat, you may be better able to make healthier choices and avoid overeating.
✓ Part of a Holistic Approach: For weight loss, it's essential to adopt a holistic approach that includes not only physical activity but also a balanced diet, proper hydration, and sufficient rest. Chair yoga can complement these lifestyle changes and contribute to an overall sense of well-being.

So, reading this book can provide you with valuable insights, guidelines, and a structured plan. Look for books that offer chair yoga routines, dietary tips, and mindfulness practices tailored to weight management. Additionally, consulting with a fitness professional or healthcare provider can help you create a personalized and effective weight loss strategy that incorporates chair yoga and other appropriate exercises. And for us, before starting your reading, it's always truly important to keep in mind that sustainable weight loss involves a combination of healthy habits and lifestyle changes, so consider chair yoga as one piece of the puzzle rather than the sole solution.

So, whether you're seeking to stay active, improve flexibility, manage stress, or simply enjoy a soothing and inclusive practice, chair yoga is here to welcome you with open arms (and a comfy chair). Embrace the journey of self-discovery and well-being as you embark on this accessible and rewarding path of chair yoga. Let's begin!

CHAPTER 1

A COMPLETE OVERVIEW OF CHAIR YOGA

n this very first chapter, we will take care of revealing a general overview of chair yoga: from how the idea was born and developed to what the fundamental principles are, we will begin to familiarize ourselves with this fantastic discipline.

Where did the idea of chair yoga come from?

If thinking about yoga makes you think of slim, flexible bodies in contortionist positions, try thinking again. Yoga has come to involve everyone and benefit everybody, regardless of age or mobility. An example is chair yoga, which is good for everyone and can really help you find (or achieve) the much-desired physical shape.

Chair yoga was originally intended for people with limited mobility, whether through trauma, disease, or age.

As we have told you in the introduction, chair yoga is a form of yoga that is adapted to be practiced while sitting on a chair or employing the chair for support. The origins of chair yoga can be traced back to the broader tradition of yoga, which originated in ancient India over 5,000 years ago. The modern concept of chair yoga, specifically tailored for individuals who may have mobility or balance challenges, is believed to have emerged in the late 20th century as a response to the needs of older adults and people with physical limitations. It was created as a way to make yoga more accessible and inclusive for those who may find it difficult to practice traditional yoga poses on the floor or a mat.

The development of chair yoga can be attributed to several yoga teachers and healthcare professionals who recognized the benefits of adapting yoga for those with limited mobility, injuries, or other health conditions. By incorporating seated poses and modifications of traditional yoga postures, chair yoga provides a gentler and more accessible approach to reaping the benefits of yoga practice.

Chair yoga has gained success in settings such as senior centers, nursing homes, workplaces, and community classes, as it offers a practical and effective way to promote physical activity, flexibility, strength, and relaxation without the need for a yoga mat or complex movements. It permits people of various skills and ages to experience the advantages of yoga and its potential to improve overall well-being.

When was chair yoga born?

Chair yoga, as a formal and distinct practice, doesn't have a specific "birth" date since it evolved gradually over time in response to the needs of individuals with limited mobility or physical challenges. However, we can trace its development to the late 20th century.

One of the pioneers credited with popularizing chair yoga is Lakshmi Voelker-Binder. In the 1980s, she began developing and teaching a form of yoga that could be practiced entirely from a chair. Her approach aimed to make yoga accessible to people with various physical limitations, including seniors, individuals with disabilities, and those recovering from injuries. Lakshmi Voelker-Binder's style of chair yoga, known as "Lakshmi Voelker Chair Yoga," gained recognition and has been used in various healthcare settings and wellness programs.

Other yoga teachers and healthcare professionals have also contributed to the development of chair yoga by creating their own adaptations and modifications of traditional yoga postures to accommodate people with different needs.

As chair yoga gained popularity, it found applications in senior centers, hospitals, rehabilitation centers, and community centers, offering a way for individuals who couldn't engage in traditional floor-based yoga to enjoy the benefits of a yoga practice. Since its inception, chair yoga has continued to evolve, and today, it remains a valuable and accessible option for people of all ages and abilities.

What exactly is chair yoga? Description and principles

Chair yoga, as we have seen so far, is a transformed form of yoga that is created to be practiced while sitting on a chair or using the chair for support. It is an accessible and soft way to obtain the benefits of yoga without having to get down on the floor or perform complex standing postures. Chair yoga incorporates various yoga poses, breathing techniques, and relaxation exercises, making it suitable for people of all ages and abilities, including those with limited mobility, balance issues, injuries, or other health conditions.

So, it's time to provide a detailed explanation of chair yoga:

Seated Postures

The primary focus of chair yoga is performing yoga poses while seated on a stable chair. These poses are adapted from traditional yoga asanas and aim to improve flexibility, strength, and balance. Participants learn how to engage their core, lengthen the spine, and move their limbs through a range of motions while seated comfortably.

Breathing Techniques

Chair yoga includes various pranayama (breath control) techniques. Participants are guided to practice deep, mindful breathing to promote relaxation, reduce stress, and increase awareness of the breath–body connection.

Gentle Stretching

The practice involves gentle stretching of different muscle groups to improve flexibility and joint mobility. The chair provides stability and support, making it safe for individuals who may find traditional stretching on the floor challenging.

Strength-Building Exercises

Participants engage in gentle strength–building movements to work on their muscles while seated. These exercises often target the upper body, lower body, and core muscles.

Balance and Stability

Chair yoga incorporates exercises to improve balance and stability. Participants can safely practice various balancing poses with the support of the chair.

Mindfulness and Meditation

Chair yoga sessions may include mindfulness practices and meditation techniques to encourage mental relaxation and inner awareness.

Relaxation and Stress Reduction

The practice emphasizes relaxation techniques, such as guided relaxation or visualization, to reduce stress, anxiety, and tension.

Accessibility

One of the main advantages of chair yoga is its inclusivity. It makes yoga accessible to individuals who might face physical limitations or difficulty with traditional yoga poses. It is commonly used in settings like senior centers, workplaces, hospitals, and rehabilitation facilities.

Customization

Chair yoga can be customized to suit the requirements and skills of the participants. Yoga instructors can modify poses and sequences based on the specific requirements of the group they are working with.

Chair yoga, as we will see in detail in the next chapter, offers numerous physical, mental, and emotional benefits, including improved flexibility, strength, posture, reduced stress, increased energy, and a sense of well-being. It is an excellent option for people looking to incorporate a gentle and mindful movement practice into their daily lives, regardless of their physical abilities or age.

The principles of chair yoga

The principles of chair yoga are based on the fundamental principles of traditional yoga, with adaptations and modifications to accommodate individuals who may have limited mobility or physical challenges. The main principles of chair yoga include:

Accessibility

Chair yoga, as we have seen, is suitable and accessible to people of all ages and skill levels. It provides a safe and comfortable way to practice yoga for those who may find it hard to deal with traditional floor-based yoga poses. The employ of a chair as a prop permits people with mobility issues, injuries, or balance concerns to participate fully in the practice.

Safety

Safety is a paramount principle in chair yoga. Poses and movements are chosen and modified to ensure that participants can practice without straining or risking injury. Yoga instructors pay close attention to proper alignment and encourage participants to listen to their bodies and practice within their individual limits.

Adaptation

Chair yoga involves adapting traditional yoga postures to be done while sitting on a chair or using the chair for support. Yoga instructors modify the poses to suit the needs and capabilities of the participants, making the practice inclusive and suitable for diverse populations.

Mindfulness

Like traditional yoga does, chair yoga emphasizes mindfulness and awareness. Everyone is encouraged to be present in the moment, be focused on their breath, and connect with their bodies and sensations during the practice.

Breath Work

Pranayama, or breath control, is an essential aspect of chair yoga. Participants learn various breathing techniques to promote relaxation, reduce stress, and enhance mental clarity.

Gentle Movement

Chair yoga focuses on soft movements that give way to flexibility, strength, and balance. The movements are slow and controlled, ensuring that participants can move comfortably within their range of motion.

Balance and Stability

Chair yoga often includes poses that are focused on balance and stability. The chair serves as a supportive prop, enabling participants to work on their balance in a safe and controlled manner.

Relaxation and Stress Reduction

Chair yoga incorporates relaxation techniques, such as guided relaxation or visualization, to help participants reduce stress and achieve a state of deep relaxation.

Individualization

Chair yoga is adaptable and can be tailored to the needs of the individuals participating in the class. Yoga instructors may modify poses, adjust sequences, and use props to create a personalized experience for each participant.

Inclusivity

Chair yoga promotes inclusivity by providing an opportunity for people with diverse abilities and backgrounds to experience the benefits of yoga. It fosters a non-judgmental and supportive environment where everyone can feel welcome and comfortable.

Overall, chair yoga embodies the essence of yoga by combining physical postures, breath work, and mindfulness in a way that is accessible, safe, and beneficial for individuals with varying levels of mobility and physical challenges.

This amazing discipline is suitable for:

✓ Elderly people
✓ Pregnant women
✓ Those with reduced mobility
✓ Wheelchair users
✓ Who has a sedentary job
✓ People who travel a lot by train, plane or car
✓ People who have suffered physical trauma and are in the recovery phase
✓ Who is overweight
✓ People with degenerative diseases
✓ Beginners
✓ People with balance problems
✓ Really everyone who wants to start yoga in a gentle way

Chair Yoga is aimed at everyone, even the most advanced practitioners. Who has never found themselves having to sit for hours? Chair yoga is suitable for a wide range of individuals and can be beneficial for various populations due to its adaptability and accessibility. But let's see more in detail.

Some of the main groups named above of people who can benefit from chair yoga include:

✓ Seniors: Chair yoga is particularly popular among seniors because it allows them to engage in a gentle form of exercise without the need to get down on the floor
✓ Individuals with Limited Mobility: Chair yoga is ideal for people with limited mobility or physical disabilities who may find traditional yoga poses challenging or impossible to perform. It provides a safe and supportive way to practice yoga and get its advantages.
✓ Office Workers: for individuals who pass long hours sitting at a desk, it can be advantageous to practice chair yoga as it helps relieve tension in the neck, shoulders, and back. It also promotes better posture and reduces the negative effects of prolonged sitting.
✓ Individuals Recovering from Injuries: Chair yoga can be used as a form of gentle exercise during the recovery phase of certain injuries. It allows individuals to maintain physical activity and flexibility while avoiding strain on injured areas.
✓ Individuals with Chronic Conditions: Chair yoga can be adapted to suit individuals with chronic health conditions such as arthritis, multiple sclerosis, fibromyalgia, or chronic pain. It gives a way to be active and manage symptoms while respecting the limitations of the condition.
✓ Beginners to Yoga: Chair yoga is an excellent starting point for those new to yoga or unsure about practicing on the floor. It introduces them to basic yoga principles and postures in a supportive and comfortable setting.
✓ Caregivers and Healthcare Professionals: Chair yoga can benefit caregivers and healthcare professionals who may experience high levels of stress and physical demands in their work. It offers them a convenient way to practice self-care and reduce stress.
✓ Busy Individuals: For those with a hectic lifestyle, chair yoga offers a convenient option for incorporating a quick and effective exercise routine into their daily schedule.

√ Pregnant Women: Chair yoga can be adapted for pregnant women, providing a gentle form of exercise and relaxation during pregnancy.
√ Mental Health and Wellness: Chair yoga's emphasis on mindfulness, relaxation, and breath work can be beneficial for individuals looking to reduce stress and anxiety and promote mental well-being.

To sum up, chair yoga is for anyone who wants to obtain the benefits of yoga in a gentle, suitable, and inclusive way. It is a versatile practice that can be tailored to suit the needs of various individuals, making it a valuable addition to many wellness and healthcare programs.

Why choose to practice chair yoga for weight loss?

We want to conclude this first descriptive chapter with a section in particular, namely the one concerning why you should choose a method, or rather a discipline, such as chair yoga, precisely with the aim of losing weight. Chair yoga, in fact, and this is why we wanted to write this specific practical guide, can be a valuable addition to a weight loss journey for several reasons, especially for individuals who may have limited mobility or physical challenges that prevent them from engaging in more vigorous forms of exercise. While chair yoga alone may not lead to relevant weight loss on its own, it can complement other healthy lifestyle changes and contribute to overall weight management. Firstly, chair yoga provides a form of physical activity that helps burn calories and contributes to a calorie deficit, which is essential for weight loss. Even though it may be low-impact, consistent chair yoga practice can gradually lead to calorie expenditure and support weight management.

Never underestimate the stress aspect when it comes to weight gain, so stress reduction can be a perfect solution. This is why stress can be a significant factor contributing to weight gain or difficulty losing weight. Chair yoga indeed incorporates relaxation techniques and mindfulness practices, which can be useful when it comes to dealing with lowering stress levels and emotional eating.

Chair yoga, as we have seen above, promotes mindfulness and awareness, which can be transferred to eating habits. Practicing mindfulness during meals can lead to more conscious eating choices, better portion control, and improved digestion.

Maybe you still don't know, but thanks to chair yoga, you can get an improved metabolism. Regular physical activity, even in the form of chair yoga, can contribute to a healthier metabolism. In addition to this, chair yoga encourages participants to connect with their bodies and become more aware of their physical sensations. This heightened body awareness may lead to recognizing hunger and fullness cues more effectively, promoting healthier eating habits.

Don't forget the strengthening core muscles factor: many chair yoga poses engage the core muscles, helping to improve core strength and stability. Stronger core muscles can support better posture and overall physical function, making it easier to engage in other physical activities.

Furthermore, chair yoga involves gentle stretching and movements that can improve flexibility and joint mobility. Enhanced flexibility makes it easier to engage in other types of exercises and physical activities, supporting a more active lifestyle.

Another important thing to consider is that chair yoga is suitable for people of all ages and abilities, including those who may be new to exercise or have limitations that prevent them from engaging in high-impact activities.

It's important to understand, as a final thought for this first chapter, that, while chair yoga can be a valuable tool in a weight loss journey, it is most effective when combined with a comprehensive approach to weight management, including a balanced and nutritious diet and other forms of physical activity, as appropriate for individual abilities and health conditions. In this way, you can accelerate weight loss even more, carry out a discipline suitable for you, who may not have much time to devote to physical activity, and regain elasticity, but above all, serenity.

CHAPTER 2

BENEFITS OF CHAIR YOGA

n the first chapter, we presented in general what chair yoga is and how it was born and developed with its principles. Let's now see what all the possible advantages that you can derive from practicing this discipline are. You will also find a short (but very short) section where possible disadvantages and contraindications will be examined. Our journey to discover chair yoga for weight loss continues!

An overall of the chair yoga advantages

Chair yoga, and this is important to repeat, is an accessible and inclusive practice suitable for people of all ages and skills, including those with lower mobility or physical challenges. So, let's see at this point what some of the many advantages of chair yoga are:

- ✓ Improved Flexibility: Chair yoga helps to increase flexibility in the joints and muscles, promoting better range of motion and reducing stiffness.
- ✓ Enhanced Strength: The practice includes gentle resistance exercises that can strengthen the muscles, particularly in the core, arms, and legs.
- ✓ Better Posture: Regular chair yoga can help improve posture and body awareness, which can be beneficial for those who spend a lot of time sitting or have back issues.
- ✓ Increased Balance: The practice often incorporates balancing poses and exercises that can help improve stability and decrease the risk of falls, which is particularly vital for seniors.
- ✓ Stress Reduction: Like traditional yoga, chair yoga includes breath work and relaxation techniques that can be useful in taking away stress and promoting overall mental well-being.
- ✓ Improved Circulation: The movements involved in chair yoga can help stimulate blood flow and circulation, benefiting cardiovascular health.
- ✓ Joint Health: Gentle movements in chair yoga can help lubricate and nourish the joints,

potentially reducing pain and discomfort associated with arthritis or other joint conditions.

✓ Enhanced Concentration and Focus: The mindful nature of chair yoga encourages participants to be present in the moment, improving focus and mental clarity.

✓ Boosted Energy Levels: Chair yoga can help combat feelings of fatigue and increase energy levels through gentle movement and deep breathing.

✓ Better Breathing: Controlled breathing exercises in chair yoga can expand lung ability and give more way to relaxation.

✓ Community and Social Interaction: Chair yoga classes furnish a supportive and inclusive environment, fostering more social interaction and a sense of community among participants.

✓ Adaptable and Accessible: Since chair yoga can be done in a seated position, it is accessible to a wide range of individuals, including those with disabilities or limited mobility.

✓ Assists Rehabilitation: Chair yoga is often used as a part of rehabilitation programs for individuals recovering from injuries or surgeries.

✓ Mind-Body Connection: Practicing chair yoga helps to strengthen the mind-body connection, fostering a deeper understanding of one's own body and its needs.

✓ Self-Care: Engaging in regular chair yoga provides individuals with an opportunity for self-care, promoting overall well-being and self-awareness.

Overall, chair yoga offers numerous physical, mental, and emotional benefits and can be a valuable addition to one's daily routine, whether as a standalone practice or in combination with other forms of exercise.

CHAIR YOGA IS SUITABLE FOR THOSE WHO DON'T HAVE TIME FOR SPORT?

We must answer this question: absolutely yes! Chair yoga can be a truly functional option for individuals who have limited time for traditional sports or exercise. One of the advantages of chair yoga is its adaptability and flexibility regarding time commitment. Many chair yoga routines can be done in short sessions, making it easier for busy individuals to incorporate them into their daily schedules. We can provide you a full list of some good reasons why chair yoga is suitable for those who don't have much time for sports:

✓ Time-Efficient: Chair yoga sessions can be as short as 10-15 minutes, and even a brief practice can offer benefits. You can choose to do a quick session in the morning, during a break at work, or before going to bed.

✓ No Commute Required: Unlike going to the gym or attending a sports class, chair yoga can be done at home, in the office, or any other convenient location. It's not so necessary to spend time traveling to a gym or studio.

✓ Accessible Throughout the Day: Since chair yoga doesn't require changing into workout clothes or taking a shower afterward, you can easily incorporate it into your daily routine without disrupting your schedule.

✓ Low Impact: As we have seen other times in this guide, chair yoga permits people to be committed to a physical activity without putting excessive strain on the body.

✓ Stress Relief and Relaxation: Even a short chair yoga session can help reduce stress,

promote relaxation, and provide mental clarity, making it a valuable tool for managing a busy schedule.
- ✓ Improved Focus and Productivity: Taking a few minutes to practice chair yoga during work or study breaks can help recharge your energy, enhance concentration, and boost productivity.
- ✓ Incorporate Mindfulness: Chair yoga incorporates mindfulness and breath work, providing a moment of mindfulness amid a busy day.
- ✓ Consistency is Key: Regular, shorter chair yoga sessions can be more sustainable and easier to stick to over time than sporadic, longer workouts.

Despite these reasons, it's always essential to take into account that even small amounts of physical activity can contribute to overall well-being. Whether you have a few minutes or more extended periods to spare, incorporating chair yoga into your daily routine can be a convenient and effective way to stay active, reduce stress, and promote a healthier lifestyle.

Is chair yoga safe? Possible contraindications

As for being a safe activity, we must affirm that chair yoga is generally considered a safe and accessible discipline, especially when compared to more physically demanding forms of yoga or exercise. It is designed to be inclusive and suitable for people of all ages, abilities, and fitness levels, including those with physical limitations or health concerns. Chair yoga instructors are trained to modify poses and sequences to accommodate individual needs and ensure safety. But even practicing it at home is a truly safe thing to do.

And, before ending this second chapter with the possible side effects, let's see some reasons why chair yoga is considered safe:

- ✓ Chair yoga involves soft movements and poses that are easy on the joints and muscles, reducing the risk of injury.
- ✓ Stability and Support: The chair provides stability and support, making it easier for participants to maintain balance and perform movements safely.
- ✓ Adaptable: Poses can be modified or customized to accommodate individual limitations, making them accessible to people with various physical conditions or mobility challenges.
- ✓ Mindful Approach: Chair yoga often emphasizes breath work and mindfulness, promoting a focus on the present moment and reducing the chances of overexertion.
- ✓ Qualified Instructors: Certified chair yoga instructors are trained to create a safe environment and provide appropriate guidance to participants, ensuring that the practice is tailored to their needs and abilities.
- ✓ Injury Prevention: Chair yoga can be used as a rehabilitative tool for those recovering from injuries or surgeries, as it allows for gentle movement without putting stress on injured areas.

However, as with any physical activity, you need to take precautions to keep in mind:

✓ Consult with a Healthcare Professional: If you have any medical conditions, injuries, or health concerns, it's essential to ask a healthcare professional before starting chair yoga or any exercise program.

✓ Listen to Your Body: It's essential to pay attention to your body and stay away from any movements or poses that cause discomfort or pain.

✓ Proper Form: Ensure that you are using the correct form and alignment during poses to minimize the risk of strain or injury.

✓ Breathing: It's essential (always remember this) to be focused on your breath and avoid holding your breath during the practice, as this can lead to tension and elevated blood pressure.

Overall, chair yoga is considered a safe and beneficial practice for most individuals, including those with limited mobility or time constraints. It can offer physical, mental, and emotional benefits, helping to improve flexibility, strength, balance, and overall well-being. If you're new to chair yoga or have specific health concerns, consider joining a class led by a certified instructor who can provide guidance and ensure a safe experience.

Chair yoga side effects and contraindications

Chair yoga, as we have just seen above, is generally safe and well-tolerated by most individuals, but like any form of physical activity, it may have some side effects and contraindications. It's essential to be aware of these potential issues and consult with a healthcare professional before starting a chair yoga practice, especially if you have any pre-existing health issues or concerns. Here are some side effects and contraindications to consider:

1. Muscle Soreness: As with any new exercise routine, you may experience mild muscle soreness, especially if you are not accustomed to physical activity. This soreness should subside within a day or two and can be managed with gentle stretching and adequate hydration.
2. Overexertion: While chair yoga is low-impact, it's still possible to overexert yourself if you push too hard or attempt poses beyond your current abilities.
3. Blood Pressure Fluctuations: Certain yoga poses and breath-work techniques may affect blood pressure. If you have high or low blood pressure, it's important to monitor how your body responds to chair yoga and inform your instructor or healthcare provider about your condition.
4. Dizziness or Lightheadedness: Some chair yoga movements involve changes in position or gentle inversions, which may cause dizziness or lightheadedness, especially if you have issues with balance or blood pressure. Be cautious when transitioning between poses and take breaks as needed.
5. Spinal troubles: people with severe spinal problems, like herniated discs or spinal fractures, should approach chair yoga with caution. Certain poses may exacerbate these conditions. Always inform your instructor about any spinal issues you have so they can provide appropriate modifications.
6. Pregnancy: While chair yoga can be beneficial for pregnant individuals, certain poses and movements may not be suitable during different stages of pregnancy.
7. Recent Surgeries or Injuries: If you've had recent surgeries or injuries, especially to

the joints, it's essential to consult with your healthcare provider before starting chair yoga to ensure that the practice won't interfere with the healing process.

8. Medical Conditions: Certain medical conditions, such as severe arthritis, osteoporosis, or other chronic health issues, may require special modifications or precautions during chair yoga. Always seek advice from your healthcare provider before beginning any exercise program.

As a final thought for this paragraph, it's always important to take into consideration that, when you are going to practice chair yoga (on your own or with instructors), you should be informed about any health conditions or concerns you may have, so an instructor can provide appropriate modifications and ensure your safety during the practice. And you can do the same! If you experience any discomfort or adverse effects during chair yoga, stop immediately and seek guidance from a healthcare professional or your instructor.

To end this chapter, we have seen that chair yoga offers numerous benefits, especially for those who need a more accessible and gentle form of exercise. Its adaptability and convenience make it an excellent choice for a diverse range of individuals, providing both physical and mental well-being. In any case, it may not be the best option for those seeking intense workouts or specific cardiovascular benefits.

CHAPTER 3

GETTING STARTED WITH CHAIR YOGA

fter having explained theoretically, in general, what chair yoga is, what its principles are, and above all, its benefits, it is time to move on to a more practical part where we will provide you with all the essential bases to be able to start in the best possible way!

How chair yoga works?

Let's start by answering this question. Chair yoga, as we have seen in the previous chapters of the book, is a modified form of yoga that is aimed at being practiced while seated on a chair or using a chair for support. It is a gentle and accessible style of yoga suitable for people of all ages and physical abilities, including those with limited mobility or balance issues.

The practice of chair yoga typically involves performing various yoga postures, stretches, breathing exercises, and relaxation techniques while seated in a stable and comfortable chair. The chair provides support and allows individuals to safely participate in yoga without having to get up and down from the floor, making it an excellent option for seniors, office workers, individuals with physical limitations, or anyone who prefers a more accessible and less strenuous form of yoga.

Despite being seated, chair yoga engages various muscle groups, encouraging strength and stability.

Practicing chair yoga can also aid in better blood flow and reduce the risk of blood pooling in the extremities. In addition to this, like other forms of yoga, chair yoga includes breathing and relaxation techniques that promote stress relief and mental well-being.

Chair yoga classes, in general, are often led by experienced instructors who provide modifications and adaptations to suit the individual needs and abilities of the participants. It can be conducted in group settings, community centers, workplaces, or even through on-line platforms, making it widely accessible to a diverse range of people. But we are talking about chair yoga at home.

This type of chair yoga is an economical and accessible way to perform yoga in the comfort of your own home. It follows the same principles and benefits as traditional chair yoga, but it is adapted to be practiced individually or with a small group of family or friends.

So, let's see in detail how home chair yoga typically works:

- ✓ Choose a Suitable Space: Find a quiet and comfortable area in your home where you can set up your chair. Be certain that there's enough room to move your arms and legs freely and that there are no obstructions.
- ✓ Select the Right Chair: Use a stable and sturdy chair without wheels. Avoid chairs with arms that restrict movement or those with an unstable structure.
- ✓ Warm-Up: Begin your practice with a gentle warm-up to prepare your body for the movements ahead. This could include neck rolls, shoulder shrugs, wrist rotations, and ankle circles.
- ✓ Chair Yoga Poses: There are numerous chair yoga poses you can explore, targeting different muscle groups and areas of the body. Some common chair yoga poses include seated twists, forward bends, side stretches, gentle back bends, and seated hip openers.
- ✓ Breathing Exercises: Integrate deep breathing exercises into your practice. These can be done while seated comfortably in the chair and are beneficial for relaxation and stress reduction.
- ✓ Mindfulness and Meditation: Include mindfulness exercises and short meditation sessions to enhance your mental focus and inner awareness.
- ✓ Cool Down and Relaxation: End your practice with a cool-down period, permitting your body to gradually relax. You can also incorporate a final relaxation pose (Savasana) where you sit comfortably, close your eyes, and focus on your breath and sensations.
- ✓ Stay Safe: While chair yoga is generally safe for most people, be careful to listen to the main signals of your body and don't take actions that may cause discomfort or pain.
- ✓ Online Resources: There are so many online resources, videos, and guided chair yoga sessions available that you can follow along with in the comfort of your home. You can find free videos on platforms like YouTube, or consider subscribing to yoga websites or apps that offer chair yoga content.

Having explained this, the beauty of home chair yoga is that you can tailor your practice to suit your individual needs, preferences, and schedule. It's a wonderful way to stay active, reduce stress, and promote overall well-being without the need for specialized equipment or a large practice space.

Necessary equipment and tools

Home chair yoga does not require any specialized equipment or tools, making it a power-ful, economical and accessible form of exercise. All you need is a sturdy and stable chair, preferably without wheels and with a straight back, to get started. It's time to show you the necessary equipment and tools for home chair yoga:

Chair

Choose a chair with a flat and firm seat, preferably without arms. This makes possible a wider range of freedom of movement during the yoga practice. Make sure the chair is stable and can support your weight comfortably.

Comfortable Clothing

Wear loose-fitting, comfortable clothing that can simplify any movement. Avoid clothing that restricts your range of motion.

Bare Feet or Non-Slip Socks

Practicing chair yoga without shoes can provide better stability and grip. If you prefer to wear socks, choose non-slip socks to prevent your feet from slipping on the chair's surface.

Optional items that can greatly improve your chair yoga practice:

- ✓ Yoga Mat: While a yoga mat is not essential for chair yoga, you may choose to place a non-slip yoga mat under your chair for added stability and to define your practice space.
- ✓ Yoga Strap: A yoga strap can be useful for certain stretches and exercises, allowing you to extend your reach and hold stretches comfortably.
- ✓ Yoga Blocks: Yoga blocks can provide additional support during some poses, helping you achieve better alignment and balance.
- ✓ Blanket or Cushion: Having a blanket or cushion nearby can be helpful for providing extra support and comfort during relaxation or seated meditation.
- ✓ Water Bottle: Stay hydrated by keeping a water bottle nearby during your practice.

And finally, we want you to always keep in mind that the essence of chair yoga is its adaptability and simplicity. You can start practicing with just a chair and your body, and if you feel the need for additional support or props, you can gradually incorporate them as you become more comfortable with the practice. The most important thing is to listen to your body, be mindful of your limitations, and enjoy the benefits of a gentle and accessible yoga practice from the comfort of your home.

How do I properly start with chair yoga?

Starting with chair yoga is a simple and enjoyable process. Follow these steps to begin your chair yoga practice at home:

1. Find a Quiet and Proper Space: What we are telling you is to look for a calm and quiet area in your home where you won't be bothered throughout your chair yoga practice.
2. Select the Right Chair: Use a sturdy and stable chair without wheels. Ensure that the chair's back is straight and the seat is flat. Avoid chairs with arms that restrict movement.
3. Wear Comfortable Clothing: Like we indicated in the previous paragraph, remove any constrictive items like belts or jewelry that might compromise your practice.
4. Warm Up: Perform some neck rolls, shoulder shrugs, wrist rotations, and ankle circles while seated in the chair.
5. Breathing Exercises: Begin your chair yoga session with some simple, deep breathing exercises. Inhale deeply through your nose, filling your belly with air, and exhale slowly through your mouth. Focus on making your breath smooth and even.
6. Learn Basic Poses: Familiarize yourself with basic chair yoga poses. Some common poses include seated twists, forward bends, side stretches, and gentle back bends. Follow along with beginner-friendly videos or guided sessions to learn these poses effectively.
7. Go at Your Own Pace: Start with simple poses and movements, gradually increasing the intensity as you gain confidence and flexibility.
8. Stay Mindful: During your practice, focus on your breath and feelings in your body. Pay attention to how each movement feels, and avoid straining or forcing yourself into uncomfortable positions.
9. Cool Down and Relaxation: End your chair yoga practice with a cool-down period to allow your body to relax. Consider a seated meditation or a few minutes of deep breathing to conclude your session.
10. Consistency is always the main thing: Aim to practice chair yoga regularly. Consistency will help you experience the cumulative benefits of the practice.
11. Seek Guidance: If you're new to chair yoga or have specific health concerns, consider attending online classes led by experienced instructors. They can provide guidance, make modifications, and ensure you're practicing safely.
12. Modify as Needed: Chair yoga can be modified to suit your individual needs and abilities. If a pose or movement feels uncomfortable, feel free to adapt it or skip it altogether.

Practicing chair yoga

Practicing chair yoga, as we have seen in the previous chapters, is a wonderful way to incorporate gentle exercise, relaxation, and mindfulness into your daily routine. So, let's now see a complete and detailed overview of how to establish and enjoy a fulfilling chair yoga practice at home:

Set Your Intentions

As the first thing to do, you can state some detailed intentions for your chair yoga practice. Consider why you want to practice chair yoga and what specific benefits you hope to achieve, such as improved flexibility, reduced stress, or better posture.

Create a suitable Space

Designate a comfortable and quiet space in your home where you can execute chair yoga exercises. Make sure there's enough room around the chair for movement and that the area promotes a sense of calm and tranquility.

Gather Your Equipment

You'll need a sturdy chair with a flat seat and no wheels. If desired, you can also use a non-slip yoga mat under the chair for added stability.

Dress Comfortably

We repeat: choose attire that doesn't restrict your range of motion.

Learn Chair Yoga Poses

Start to put yourself in a variety of chair yoga poses that are focused on different areas of the body. Some common poses include:

1. Seated Twist: Twist your torso gently to the right and left, holding onto the chair's backrest for support.
2. Forward Bend: Slowly hinge forward from your hips while keeping your back straight and your hands on your thighs or reaching toward your feet.
3. Side Stretch: Reach one arm overhead and lean to the opposite side, creating a gentle stretch along the torso.
4. Gentle Back Bend: Arch your spine slightly backward while supporting your lower back with your hands.
5. Seated Hip Opener:
6. Mindful Movement: As you flow through the poses, maintain mindfulness by focusing on your breath and sensations. Avoid rushing and pay attention to your body's feedback.

Modify for Comfort

Change the poses to adapt them to your individual needs and limitations. Feel free to use props like a yoga strap or blocks to enhance your practice.

Cool Down and Relaxation

End your chair yoga practice with a cool-down period to allow your body to relax. Consider practicing seated meditation or a guided relaxation exercise.

Practice Regularly

Aim for consistency in your chair yoga practice. Even little sessions of 10-15 minutes can be beneficial. Practicing regularly will help you experience the cumulative benefits of the practice.

Online Resources

Utilize online platforms for guided chair yoga classes or follow along with instructional videos to learn new poses and sequences.

Enjoy the Process

Embrace the journey of chair yoga and savor the physical and mental benefits it brings. Celebrate your progress and the improvements you notice over time.

To conclude this third chapter, we must say that chair yoga is about making the practice accessible and enjoyable for you. It's an excellent way to stay active, promote relaxation, and cultivate a deeper mind-body connection from the comfort of your own home.

It can also be a gentle and effective way to improve flexibility, strength, and overall well-being while enjoying the convenience of practicing at home (or work). As you become more comfortable with chair yoga, you can explore new poses and variations to keep your practice fresh and engaging.

Also take into account that chair yoga is a flexible practice that can be tailored to meet different fitness levels and health conditions.

CHAPTER 4

HOW TO APPROACH THE 28-DAY CHALLENGE FOR MAXIMAL RESULTS

ere we are at another practical part that interests us even more closely: the famous challenge that will allow us, thanks to chair yoga, to lose weight, have a better physical shape, and make us feel better about ourselves, as well as have a better self-esteem. Let's begin!

Chair yoga tips for obtaining general maximal results

Chair yoga is a great option, as we have already seen, for individuals who have mobility issues or find it challenging to practice traditional yoga on a mat. To obtain general maximal results from chair yoga, consider the following tips:

- ✓ Consistency: Like any practice or wellness routine, consistency is the main thing (never forget it). Aim to incorporate chair yoga into your daily routine or at least a few times per week to see noticeable improvements over time.
- ✓ Proper Posture: focus on maintaining your posture during chair yoga poses to maximize the advantages and avoid any strain.
- ✓ Breathing Techniques: Practice deep, mindful breathing throughout the chair yoga session. Deep breathing can be so useful for lowering stress, increasing oxygen intake, and enhancin the relaxation response.
- ✓ Full Range of Motion: Pay attention to moving through the full range of motion for each pose. This will help improve flexibility and joint mobility.
- ✓ Strength-Building Poses: add strength-building poses into your routine to move different muscle groups. For example, practice seated leg lifts, arm circles, or chest openers.
- ✓ Balance Exercises: Include balance exercises that challenge your stability. Holding onto the back of the chair lightly, try lifting one foot off the ground and holding the position for a few seconds. Alternate between legs.

✓ Modify as Needed: Don't be afraid to modify the poses to suit your individual needs and abilities. Your chair can be used as a support for various standing poses as well.
✓ Mindfulness and Meditation: End your chair yoga practice with some mindfulness or meditation.
✓ Warm-Up and Cool-Down: Always begin your chair yoga session with a gentle warm-up to prepare your body for movement. Similarly, end with a cool-down to allow your body to get relaxed and recovered.
✓ Seek Guidance: If you're new to chair yoga or have specific health concerns, consider joining a chair yoga class led by a qualified instructor. They can guide you through the poses safely and provide modifications tailored to your needs.

Chair yoga: tips for obtaining maximal weight loss and maximal results

While chair yoga can provide numerous health benefits, it can also be an effective form of exercise for weight loss. Weight loss - remember this important concept - primarily depends on creating a calorie deficit, which means burning more calories than you consume. While chair yoga can contribute to burning some calories, it may not be enough to result in significant weight loss on its own.

In any case, if you enjoy chair yoga and want to incorporate it into your weight loss journey, you can combine it with other lifestyle changes to maximize results. So, it's time to show you some very useful tips about it:

BALANCED DIET

Focus on a balanced and healthy diet that includes a variety of nutrient-dense foods. Decrease your amount of sugary, processed, and high-calorie foods. Portion control is essential for weight loss.

REGULAR PHYSICAL ACTIVITY

Chair yoga can be complemented with other forms of physical activity that are more intensive and calorie-burning. Based on your fitness level, you can incorporate activities like walking, swimming, cycling, or aerobics.

STRENGTH TRAINING

Join in some strength-training exercises in your chair yoga session. Building muscle mass can boost your metabolism and be useful for weight loss. You can employ light dumbbells or resistance bands during chair yoga or perform separate strength workouts.

If possible, try to increase the intensity and duration of your chair yoga sessions. Challenge yourself with more advanced poses or increase the number of repetitions for strength-building exercises.

Monitor Progress

Check your progress through a food diary, tracking physical activity, and noting any changes in weight or body measurements. This will help you stay committed and make the necessary adjustments to your routine.

Stay Hydrated

Drink a large amount of water during the day. Staying hydrated can help control overeating.

Consistency

As with any weight-loss plan, consistency is crucial. Stick to your chair yoga practice and other physical activities, as well as a healthy diet, for long-term results.

Anyway, despite these tips, it's always important to take into account that weight loss is a gradual process, and it's essential to approach it with a holistic approach that includes both physical activity and a healthy diet. Chair yoga can be a valuable addition to an overall weight loss plan, contributing to improved flexibility, muscle tone, and overall well-being.

Chair yoga for losing belly fat

While chair yoga can be a relevant to achieve for a general weight loss, it's important to note that spot reduction (targeting fat loss in a specific area, such as the belly) is generally not effective. To lose belly fat, you need to pay more attention to overall fat loss through a match of regular exercise, a balanced diet, and lifestyle changes. However, adding chair yoga to your fitness routine can still be advantageous for your overall health and well-being.

But let's see some good ways chair yoga can contribute to your fitness and weight loss journey:

✓ Expanded Physical Activity: Chair yoga, as we have known so far, is all about gentle movements that can help increase your overall physical activity level. Every bit of movement counts towards burning calories, which can contribute to the calorie deficit needed for fat loss.
✓ Stress Decreasing: Chronic stress can be one of the main reasons for weight gain, especially in the abdominal area. Chair yoga often incorporates mindfulness and relaxation techniques, which can help reduce stress levels and potentially support weight loss efforts.

✓ Improved Metabolism: While chair yoga may not significantly increase your metabolic rate compared to more intense exercises, it can still play a role in maintaining muscle mass and supporting your overall metabolism.
✓ Better Digestion: Certain chair yoga poses can aid in improving digestion and reducing bloating, which may contribute to a flatter belly appearance.
✓ Enhanced Flexibility and Mobility: Chair yoga can help improve flexibility and mobility, making it easier to engage in other forms of exercise that can aid in weight loss.
✓ Core Strengthening: Some chair yoga poses target the core muscles. Targeting this area can be essential when it comes to improving the tone and strength of the abdominal area.
✓ To maximize the effects of chair yoga for overall weight loss, consider combining it with other forms of exercise and lifestyle changes:
✓ Cardiovascular Exercise: Incorporate regular cardiovascular exercises like walking, jogging, cycling, or swimming to help burn calories and support fat loss.
✓ Strength Training: this type of training exercise is fundamental to building muscle. More muscles are responsible for boosting your resting metabolic rate and contributing to fat burning.
✓ Balanced Diet: be committed to a varied, balanced and nutritious diet that gets a variety of whole foods, lean proteins, fruits, vegetables, and healthy fats. Control your portion sizes and be careful about your calorie intake.
✓ Hydration: Stay well-hydrated throughout the day by drinking lots of water, which can support overall health and may help control appetite.
✓ Consistency: Consistency, and we will never be so tired to repeat it, is key to achieving any fitness or weight loss goal. Set realistic goals and stick to your exercise and diet plans.

And finally, losing belly fat and achieving overall weight loss require a global approach that involves a combination of exercise, diet, and lifestyle changes.

Chair yoga for body recomposition

Chair yoga can be a helpful component of a body recomposition plan that involves simultaneously reducing body fat and building or maintaining muscle mass. While chair yoga may not provide the same level of intensity as traditional strength training exercises, it can still contribute to body recomposition by improving flexibility and mobility and promoting relaxation, which can aid in stress management and recovery.

Let's see at this point in the book how you can incorporate chair yoga into your body recomposition routine:

✓ Include Strength-Building Poses: Although chair yoga focuses on gentle movements, certain poses can still engage and strengthen various muscle groups. Poses like seated leg lifts, seated twists, and chair squats can help target specific muscles and contribute to body recomposition.
✓ Integrate Balance Exercises: Balancing poses, even while using the chair for support, can engage your core and leg muscles. Try exercises like one-legged seated balance or standing on one foot while holding onto the back of the chair lightly.
✓ Mindful Breathing: Be more focused on your breath during chair yoga. Deep, controlled

breathing can engage the core muscles and promote relaxation, which can aid in stress reduction and overall well-being.
- ✓ Focus on Flexibility: Improving flexibility is essential for a well-rounded fitness routine. Chair yoga can help you stretch and lengthen various muscle groups, promoting better mobility and range of motion.
- ✓ Use Chair Yoga for Active Recovery: On rest days or after more intense workouts, consider incorporating chair yoga as a form of active recovery. It can help ease muscle tension, reduce soreness, and improve blood circulation.
- ✓ Consistency and Variety: Like any fitness routine, consistency is key. Aim to practice chair yoga regularly, but don't solely rely on it. Incorporate other forms of exercise like cardiovascular activities and strength training to achieve a balanced approach to body recomposition.
- ✓ Nutrition: diet is fundamental when it comes to dealing with body recomposition. As we have already said, follow a balanced and nutritious diet to reach your fitness goals.
- ✓ Monitor Progress: Keep track of your body's recomposition progress over time. Take measurements, take photos, or use other methods to track changes in body composition and strength.

As a final thought, before moving on to the approach of utilizing chair yoga for your weight loss, you should always take into account that, while chair yoga can be a valuable addition to your body recomposition plan, it's essential to acknowledge that more intense forms of exercise, such as resistance training, are typically more effective for building and maintaining muscle mass. For optimal results, consider combining chair yoga with other forms of exercise that target various muscle groups and challenge your body in different ways.

How to properly approach a 28-day chair yoga challenge

Approaching a 28-day chair yoga challenge can be a wonderful and functional way to obtain what we have talked about so far in this book: flexibility, strength, and overall well-being. Let's look at a suggested approach:

- ✓ Set Clear Goals: establish what you want to obtain through this challenge. Having clear goals will be truly important for keeping you motivated.
- ✓ Find a Chair Yoga Program: Look for a reputable chair yoga program or challenge that offers a structured sequence of daily or weekly sessions. There are so many online resources and apps that might pose such challenges.
- ✓ Start Slowly: If you're new to yoga or have any health concerns, begin at a comfortable pace. Gradually ease into the practice to avoid strain or injury.
- ✓ Schedule Regular Practice: Commit to practicing chair yoga regularly throughout the 28 days. Consistency is key to seeing progress.
- ✓ Create a Supportive Environment: Set up a quiet and comfortable space to practice, free from distractions.
- ✓ Listen to Your Body: Always be careful of how your body feels during the practice. Modify poses or take breaks if necessary.

✓ Stay Hydrated: Drinking plenty of water to stay hydrated is always vital, especially if you're engaging in physical activity.
✓ Track Your Progress: Keep a journal or use an app to track your daily practice and note any improvements you observe.
✓ Stay Positive and Patient: Progress may vary from day to day. Stay positive and patient with yourself throughout the challenge.
✓ Celebrate Achievements: Be conscious and celebrate your accomplishments, no matter how little they may seem. Completing a 28-day challenge is an achievement in itself!

And, as a final indication, keep in mind that chair yoga is designed to be accessible for various fitness levels and can be a wonderful way to promote relaxation and well-being.

A 28-day chair yoga challenge

A 28-day chair yoga challenge can be a fantastic way to enhance your flexibility, strength, and overall well-being. So, at this point, we want to suggest a very useful plan for the chair yoga challenge:

WEEK 1: FOUNDATIONS OF CHAIR YOGA

✓ Day 1: Introduction to Chair Yoga and basic seated stretches.
✓ Day 2: Gentle neck and shoulder stretches.
✓ Day 3: Seated twists and torso stretches.
✓ Day 4: Hip and thigh stretches in the chair.
✓ Day 5: Practice deep breathing and relaxation techniques.
✓ Day 6: Review and rest day.
✓ Day 7: Full-body chair yoga flow.

WEEK 2: BUILDING STRENGTH AND BALANCE

✓ Day 8: Chair squats and leg exercises.
✓ Day 9: Arm and upper body strength poses.
✓ Day 10: Focus on core muscles while seated.
✓ Day 11: Balancing poses with the support of the chair.
✓ Day 12: Practice mindfulness and meditation.
✓ Day 13: Review and rest day.
✓ Day 14: Full-body chair yoga flow incorporating strength and balance.

WEEK 3: DEEPENING THE PRACTICE

✓ Day 15: Explore seated forward bends and stretches.
✓ Day 16: Open up the chest and improve posture.
✓ Day 17: Gentle back bends and heart-opening poses.
✓ Day 18: Focus on seated hip openers.

✓ Day 19: Practice mindfulness and meditation.
✓ Day 20: Review and rest day.
✓ Day 21: Full-body chair yoga flow with deeper stretches.

✓ Day 22: Practice restorative poses with the chair.
✓ Day 23: Guided relaxation and breathing exercises.
✓ Day 24: Gentle flows to integrate what you've learned.
✓ Day 25: Mindfulness and meditation practice.
✓ Day 26: Review and rest day.
✓ Day 27: Full-body chair yoga flow with a focus on relaxation.
✓ Day 28: Celebration and reflection on your chair yoga journey.

It's always important to remind yourself to warm up before each session, listen to your body, and modify poses if needed. Set aside a specific time each day for your practice, and if you miss a day, don't worry; just pick up where you left off. Embrace the challenge and the pros that chair yoga can bring to your life!

Approaching a 28-day weight loss challenge

Ultimately, we want to show you how to approach a specific chair yoga weight loss challenge!

One of the main causes of weight gain is overeating. Chair yoga can help combat this problem by increasing body awareness. During the practice, it is important to focus on the feeling of satiety in the body to avoid eating more than necessary.

Sitting for many hours a day at work or at home can affect health and movement, often leading to weight gain. However, chair yoga can be a great exercise to keep the body moving and aid in weight loss. This practice involves using the chair as a point of support to perform certain yoga positions with the support of the legs and arms to strengthen muscles and improve posture. While it doesn't involve a high calorie burn, it helps to increase flexibility and control of your body.

Furthermore, chair yoga can help reduce stress, which can lead to increased food intake due to anxiety or depression.

In addition to increasing body awareness, chair yoga can also help burn calories. While you won't burn as many calories as with a high-intensity workout, chair yoga can help tone your muscles and increase muscle strength. If you build more muscles, you will be able to burn calories while resting, too. Additionally, chair yoga can help improve posture and flexibility, which can lead to an increase in overall physical activity and therefore the ability to burn more calories.

Embarking on a 28-day chair yoga challenge for weight loss can be a beneficial and sustainable way to incorporate physical activity into your routine. Let's see, even here, a suggested approach tailored toward weight loss:

Week 1: Establishing the Practice

✓ Day 1: Introduction to Chair Yoga and basic seated stretches to get acquainted with the practice.
✓ Day 2: Gentle neck and shoulder stretches to release tension.
✓ Day 3: Seated twists and torso stretches to engage the core.
✓ Day 4: Hip and thigh stretches in the chair to target lower body muscles.
✓ Day 5: Practice deep breathing and relaxation techniques to manage stress, which can impact weight loss.
✓ Day 6: Review and rest day to allow your body to recover.
✓ Day 7: Full-body chair yoga flow to start integrating movements.

Week 2: Increasing Intensity

✓ Day 8: Chair squats and leg exercises to work on lower body strength.
✓ Day 9: Arm and upper body strength poses to engage the arms and shoulders.
✓ Day 10: Focus on the core muscles while seated to strengthen and tone the midsection.
✓ Day 11: Balancing poses with the support of the chair to challenge stability and core strength.
✓ Day 12: Practice mindfulness and meditation to support mental well-being during weight loss.
✓ Day 13: Review and rest day to give your body time to recuperate.
✓ Day 14: Full-body chair yoga flow incorporating strength and balance.

Week 3: Intensifying the Practice

✓ Day 15: Explore seated forward bends and stretches to promote flexibility.
✓ Day 16: Open up the chest and improve posture to enhance body awareness.
✓ Day 17: Gentle back bends and heart-opening poses to stretch and strengthen the back.
✓ Day 18: Focus on seated hip openers to increase mobility in the hips and lower body.
✓ Day 19: Practice mindfulness and meditation to continue fostering a positive mindset.
✓ Day 20: Review and rest day to allow your body to recover.
✓ Day 21: Full-body chair yoga flow with deeper stretches.

Week 4: Boosting Calorie Burn and Relaxation

✓ Day 22: Practice restorative poses with the chair to aid relaxation and recovery.
✓ Day 23: Guided relaxation and breathing exercises to face stress and get more well-being.
✓ Day 24: Gentle flows to integrate what you've learned and continue burning calories.
✓ Day 25: Mindfulness and meditation practice to support your weight loss journey.
✓ Day 26: Review and rest day to give your body time to recuperate.

✓ Day 27: Full-body chair yoga flow with a focus on relaxation and mindfulness.
✓ Day 28: Celebration and reflection on your chair yoga journey for weight loss.

How much time should I devote to this type of yoga per day to get results?

To achieve significant results with yoga, you need to devote at least 30 minutes a day to the practice. However, the optimal time varies based on your level of experience and the kind of activity you choose. For beginners, the best idea is to begin with sessions of 15–20 minutes a day and gradually increase the duration. For experts, on the other hand, it can even be up to an hour per day of practice. Consistency in practice is also important, rather than an intense but sporadic session.

The optimal duration for a yoga practice varies according to the level of experience and the type of yoga. It is recommended that you dedicate at least 30 minutes a day, but beginners can start with 15–20 minutes and build up gradually. Consistency in practice is more important than intense but sporadic duration.

As a final tip, it's always truly important for us to make you aware of the fact that chair yoga alone may not be the only factor contributing to weight loss. Be patient with yourself, as weight loss is a gradual process. Enjoy the challenge and the positive impact it can have on your overall well-being!

And that concludes an important part of our book. In the following chapters, we'll start showing you real exercises that will actually help you reach your weight loss goal.

CHAPTER 5

CHAIR YOGA EXERCISES

ere we are at another really fundamental part that concerns our topic: real yoga exercises, or rather, chair yoga! We have seen so far that this form of yoga is based on postures performed through the use of a chair, which allows you to maintain an adequate position while working on muscle strength, flexibility and breathing. Thanks to targeted exercises, you can also burn calories and achieve your goal of losing weight. From here on, we will begin to provide you with detailed instructions on how to carry out these exercises. For each of these exercises, there will also be a specific explanation regarding weight loss. Get ready as we start with the real action!

Chair Spinal Twist

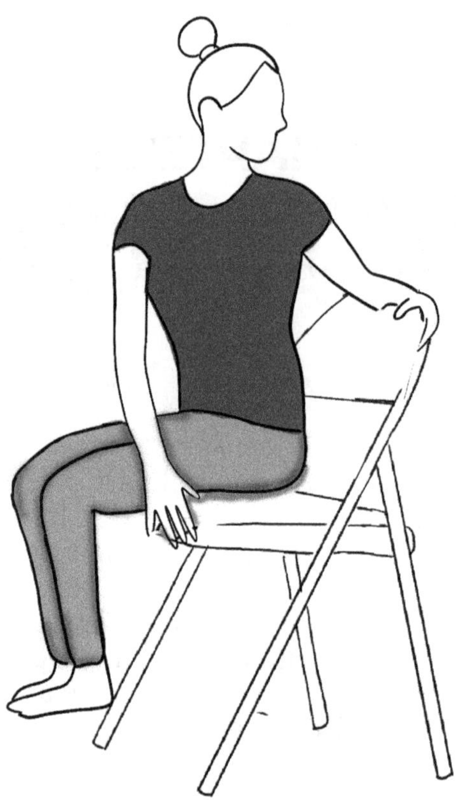

Chair spinal yoga is a modified form of yoga that focuses on gentle stretches and movements to promote flexibility and relaxation in the spine while sitting on a chair. Before starting any of these exercises, always keep in mind to move slowly and mindfully, paying more attention to your breath and never forcing any movement. In any case, chair spinal yoga is a gentle practice suitable for people with mobility issues or those who spend long hours sitting at a desk.

Here's a detailed explanation of some chair spinal yoga exercises:

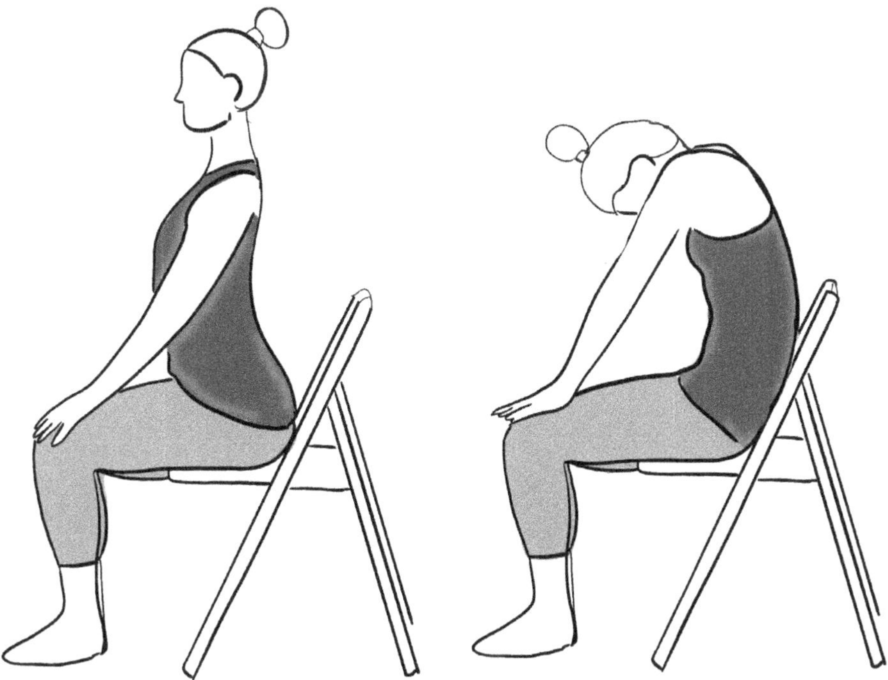

Sit upright on the chair with your feet flat on the floor and your hands on your knees. Inhale, arch your back, and lift your chest (Cow pose). Exhale, round your back, and tuck your chin (Cat pose). Repeat this flow gently for a few breaths. Below, we will explain in detail:

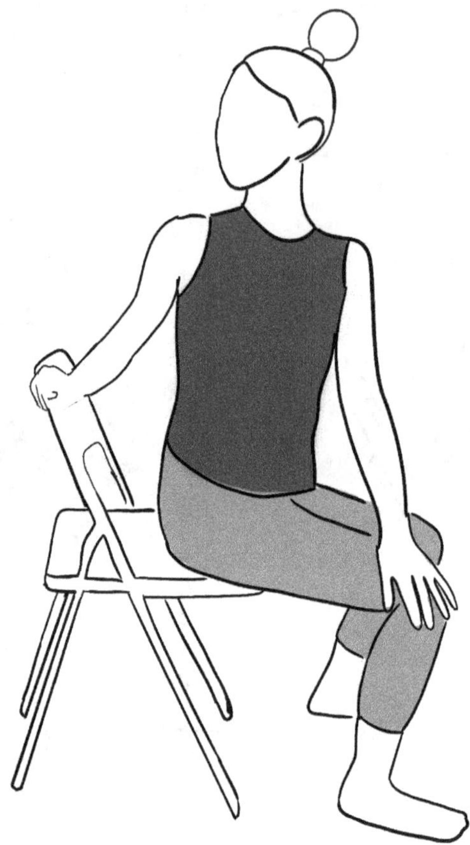

To perform a seated twist in yoga, follow these steps:

- ✓ Sit on the floor with your legs extended straight in front of you.
- ✓ Bend your right knee and put your right foot on the outside of your left thigh, close to your left knee.
- ✓ Keep your left leg extended and firmly grounded on the floor.
- ✓ Inhale, lengthen your spine, and sit tall.
- ✓ As you exhale, twist your torso to the right, bringing your left hand to the outside of your right knee.
- ✓ Place your right hand behind you for support, keeping your spine straight.
- ✓ Use each inhale to lengthen your spine and each exhale to gently deepen the twist.
- ✓ Hold the twist for a few little breaths and note the stretch along your spine and in your abdomen.
- ✓ To release, inhale and untwist back to the center.
- ✓ Do the twist on the other side, bending your left knee and twisting to the left.

It's essential to remember to maintain a comfortable and steady breath throughout the pose and avoid forcing the twist beyond your comfort level.

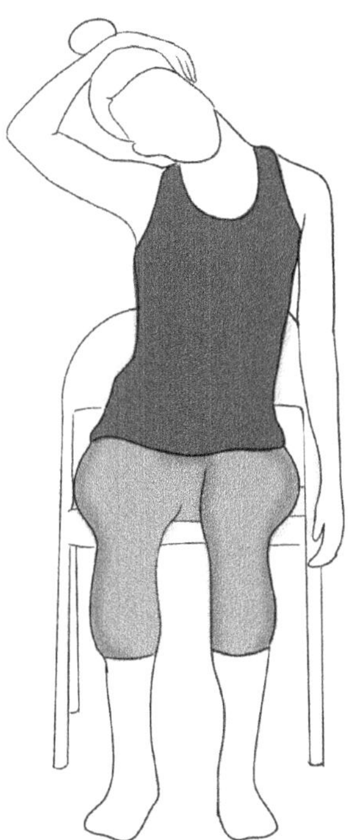

Let's see some chair yoga neck stretches that you can try:

✓ Neck Rolls: Sit up straight in your chair and gently roll your head in a circular motion, bringing your ear towards your shoulder, then the back of your head, then the other ear, and finally the front of your neck. Repeat in both clockwise and counterclockwise directions.
✓ Neck Tilts: While sitting tall, tilt your head to one side, bringing your ear towards your shoulder. Hold for a few seconds, and then repeat on the other side.
✓ Chin Tucks: Keep your spine straight and slowly tuck your chin towards your chest, feeling a stretch in the back of your neck. Hold for a few seconds, and then release.
✓ Neck Stretch with Arm Reach: Sit tall and extend one arm out to the side. Take your opposite hand and gently grasp the top of your head, then slowly tilt your head to the side, feeling a stretch along the side of your neck and shoulder. Do the same on the other side.
✓ Shoulder Shrugs: Raise your shoulders towards your ears and hold for a few seconds, then relax and let them drop. Repeat a few times to release tension in your neck and shoulders.

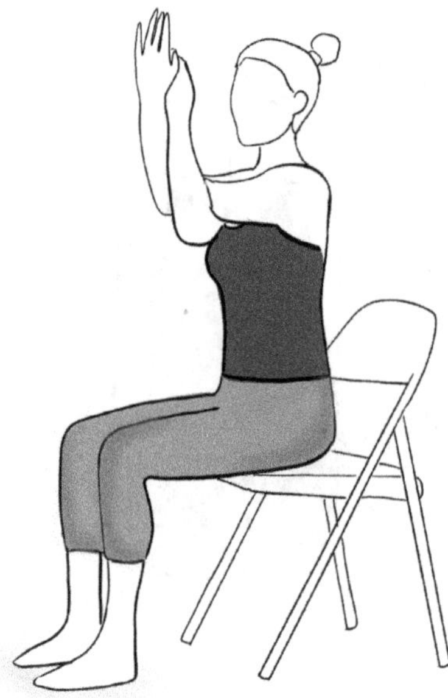

The seated spinal twist with Eagle arms is a variation of the traditional seated twist that incorporates Eagle arms, providing an added shoulder stretch. Here's how you can do it:

✓ Begin by sitting on the floor with your legs placed straight in front of you.
✓ Bend your right knee and place your right foot on the outside of your left thigh, close to your left knee, just like in the regular seated twist.
✓ Next, cross your left arm over your right arm in front of your chest. Bend both elbows and try to bring the palms of your hands together. If your palms don't touch, you can simply bring the backs of your hands together or hold them in the direction of the opposite shoulders.
✓ Inhale, lengthen your spine, and sit tall.
✓ As you exhale, twist your torso to the right, bringing your Eagle arms to the outside of your right knee. Your right hand should be closer to your body, and your left hand should be closer to your knee.
✓ Use the pressure of your arms against your knee to deepen the twist.
✓ Turn your head to look over your right shoulder, maintaining the eagle arm position.
✓ Keep the twist for some breaths, feeling the stretch along your spine, shoulders, and upper back.
✓ To release, inhale and untwist back to the center, and then release the Eagle arms.
✓ Repeat the twist on the other side, bending your left knee and twisting to the left while crossing the right arm over the left with the Eagle arms.

As always, listen to your body and practice the pose within your comfortable range of motion. If you're new to this variation or have any concerns,

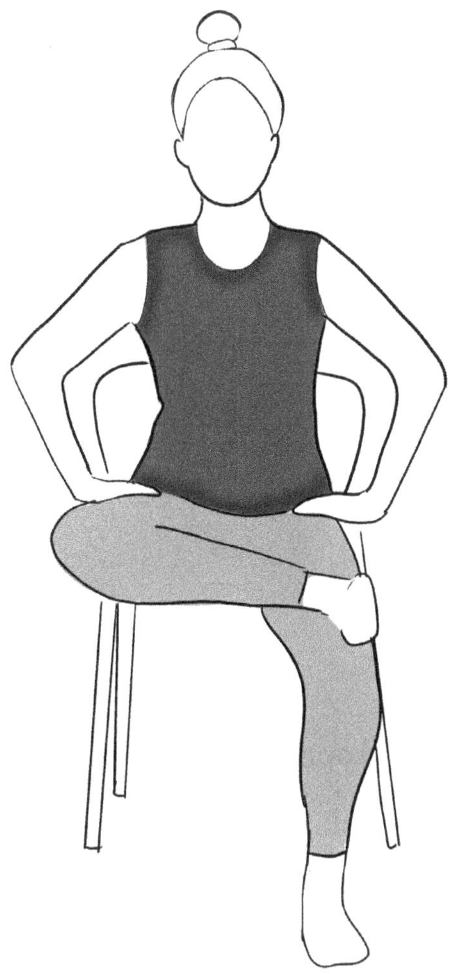

Seated Pigeon Pose is a yoga pose that can be done in a chair, making it suitable for those who may have difficulty with traditional yoga positions. Let's also see how to do this chair yoga position:

✓ Sit on a chair with your feet flat on the floor and your spine straight.
✓ Put your right ankle on top of your left knee. You should obtain a figure-four shape with your legs.
✓ Flex your right foot to preserve your knee. You can also gently press your right hand against your right knee to stabilize the position.
✓ Stay in this position and gently lean forward from your hips, keeping your back straight.
✓ Maintain the stretch for about 15–30 seconds while breathing deeply.
✓ To release the pose, slowly sit back up and place both feet on the floor.
✓ Repeat the same steps with your left ankle on top of your right knee to stretch the other side.

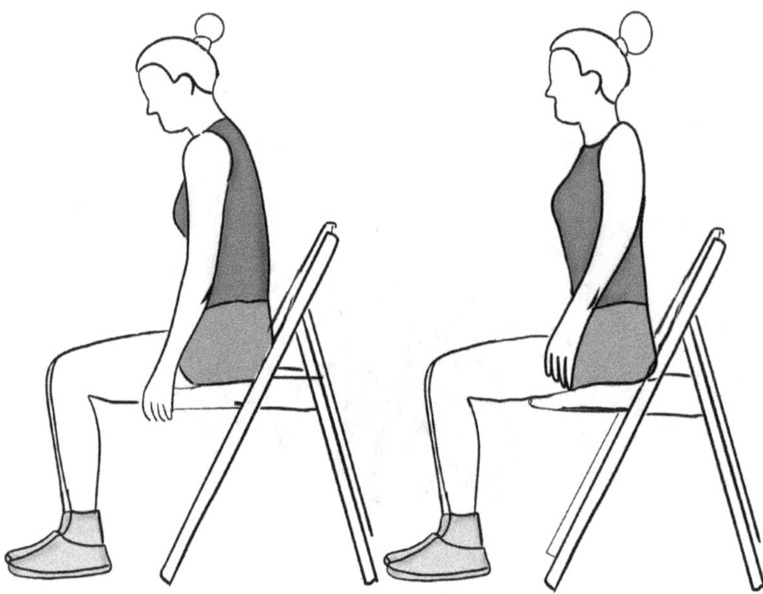

As we have already seen, it is a useful option for those with limited mobility or who prefer to practice seated exercises. So, let's see how to add yoga to your daily routine and promote overall well-being. Here's how to do shoulder rolls:

✓ Sit comfortably on a chair with your feet flat on the floor, hip-width apart, and your hands resting on your thighs.
✓ Inhale and lift your shoulders up toward your ears, tensing them gently.
✓ As you exhale, roll your shoulders back and down in a smooth circular motion. Imagine drawing circles with your shoulder blades.
✓ Continue the circular motion for a few rounds, making sure to keep the movement slow and controlled.
✓ After a few rounds in one direction, switch and roll your shoulders to the opposite side.
✓ Throughout the exercise, maintain relaxed breathing and focus on the sensation in your shoulders. If you notice any discomfort or pain, lower the size of the circles or omit the exercise if necessary. The goal is to release tension and create more mobility in the shoulder joints.
✓ Repeat this movement several times.

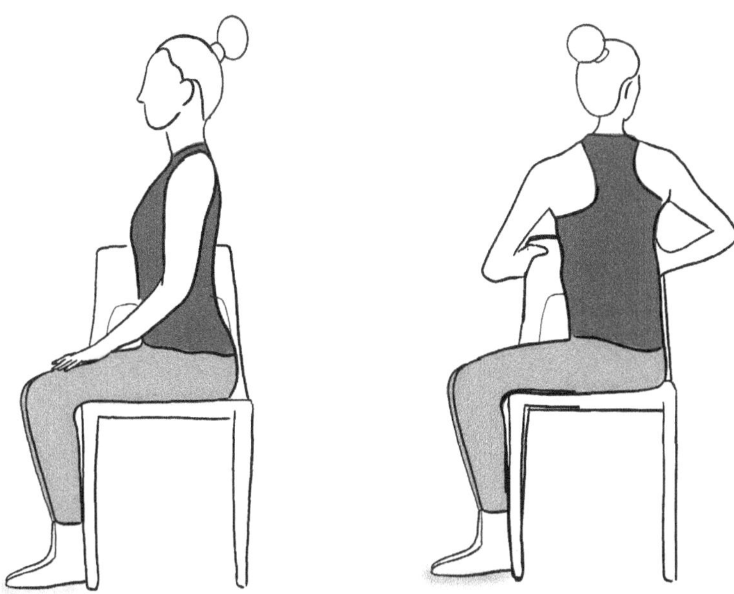

Chair yoga spinal twists can be a beneficial addition to your weight loss journey as they help to improve digestion, stimulate the abdominal organs, and increase blood flow to the area. While chair yoga alone may not be the sole factor in weight loss, it can complement a balanced diet and regular exercise routine. Let's see in detail a simple chair yoga spinal twist you can try:

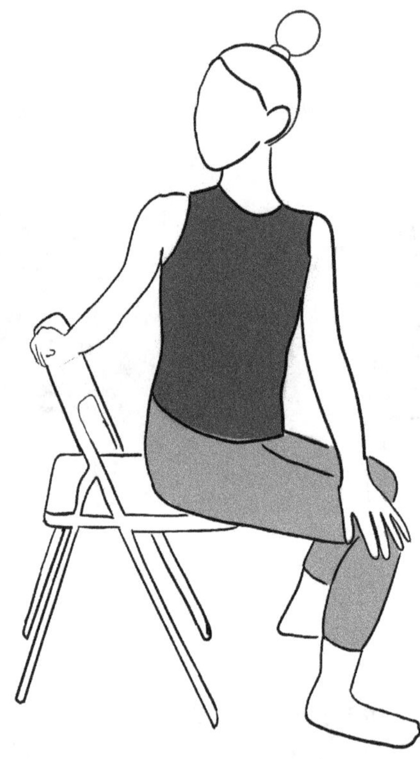

✓ Place yourself on a chair with your feet flat on the floor and your hands resting on your thighs.
✓ Inhale deeply, lengthening your spine, and exhale to prepare for the twist.
✓ As you inhale, lift your right arm up towards the ceiling, lengthening your spine even more.
✓ Exhale and gently twist to the right, bringing your left hand to the outside of your right knee or the armrest of the chair.
✓ Use each inhale to lengthen your spine and each exhale to deepen the twist slightly. Keep your shoulders relaxed and stay away from any strain.
✓ Keep the twist for a few breaths, feeling the light compression in the abdominal area.
✓ Inhale to release the twist, and then do the same on the other side, lifting your left arm up and twisting to the left.
✓ Continue alternating sides for a few rounds.

Shoulder Seated

Chair yoga shoulder seated seems to be a combination of chair yoga and seated shoulder exercises. Below is a detailed explanation of a chair yoga routine that specifically targets the shoulders while remaining seated:

Shoulder Rolls

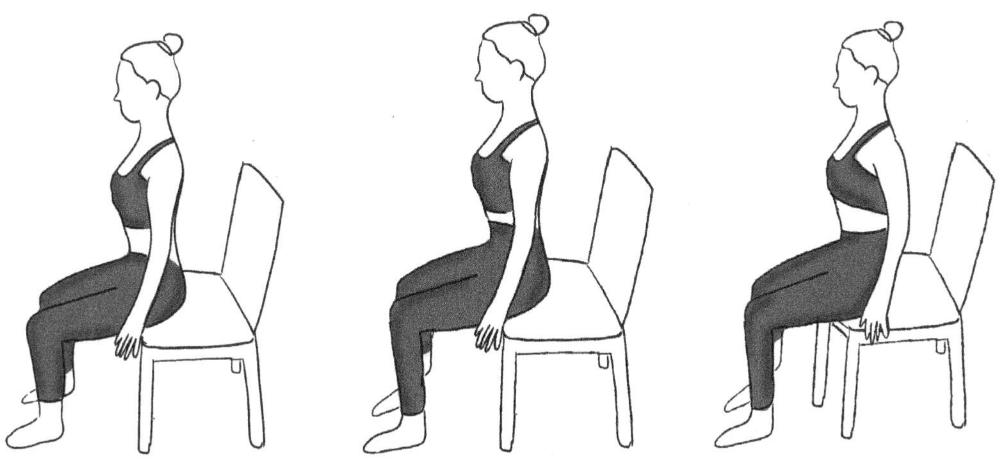

Sit on a chair with your feet flat on the floor and your hands on your thighs.

Inhale deeply and lift your shoulders up towards your ears. Exhale and roll your shoulders back and down in a smooth circular motion. Repeat this movement several times, allowing your shoulder blades to move freely.

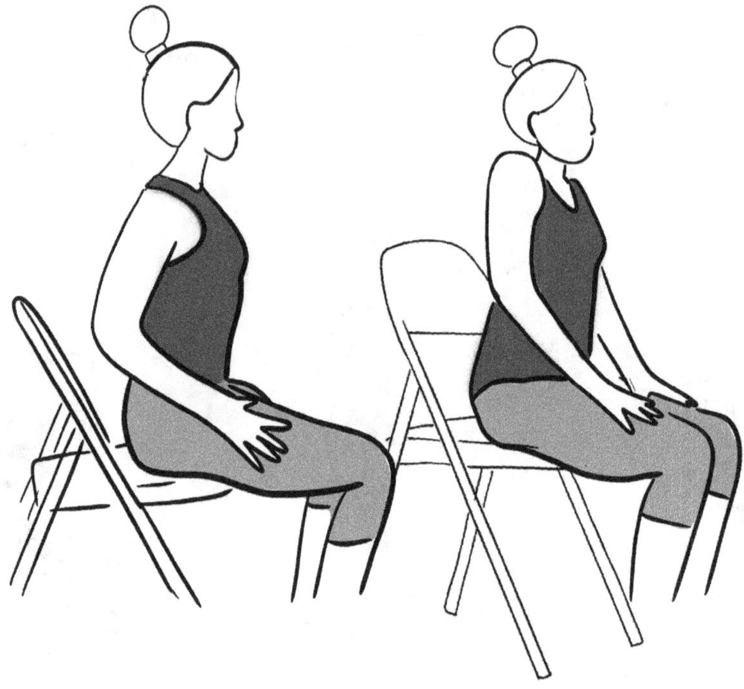

Chair yoga shoulder shrugs are another amazing way to release tension in the shoulders and upper back. Here's how to do it:

✓ Sit comfortably on a chair. In this case, your feet must be flat on the floor, and your hands must be on your thighs or on the armrests of the chair.
✓ Inhale deeply, and as you exhale, lift your shoulders up towards your ears, tensing them.
✓ Hold the tension in your shoulders for a brief moment.
✓ As you inhale, release the tension and let your shoulders drop back to their relaxed position.
✓ Repeat the shoulder shrug movement for several rounds, coordinating your breath with the movement.

The key to this exercise is to be mindful of the tension in your shoulders as you lift them and the relaxation as you release them back down. It's a functional way to eliminate built-up stress and tightness in the shoulder area.

You can perform chair yoga shoulder shrugs throughout the day, especially if you spend long hours sitting at a desk or in front of a computer. It helps prevent stiffness and promotes better circulation in the shoulder region. Remember to maintain slow and controlled movements to avoid any strain.

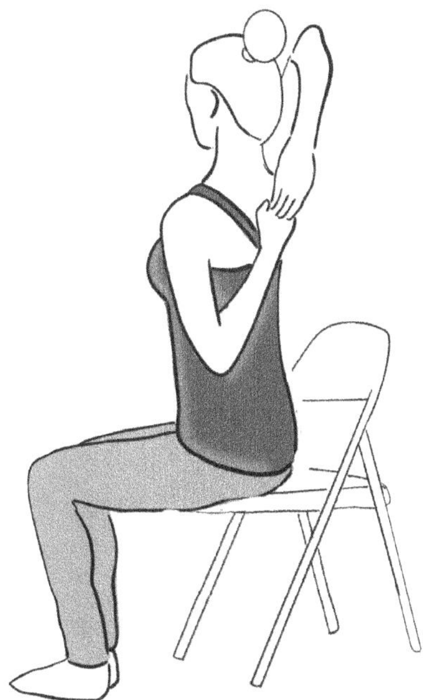

Seated cow-face arms are another good way to take away the tension from the shoulders and improve flexibility in the upper body. It's a beneficial pose, especially if you spend a lot of time sitting at a desk or engaging in activities that may cause shoulder tightness.

Seated Cow Face Arms, in fact, is a yoga pose that stretches and opens the shoulders and upper arms. Here's how to do it:

✓ Sit on the floor or on a chair. Remember to have a totally straight back.
✓ Extend your right arm out to the side at shoulder level, parallel to the ground.
✓ Angle your right elbow and reach your right hand behind your head, aiming to be in contact with the upper back.
✓ Now, bring your left arm out to the side as well, also at shoulder level and parallel to the ground.
✓ Angle your left elbow and reach your left hand behind your back, aiming to touch your right hand.
✓ The posture should resemble the shape of crossed arms behind your back, with the right elbow pointing up and the left elbow pointing down. The goal is to have the hands meet between the shoulder blades.
✓ Hold the position for a few breaths, gently stretching and opening the shoulders.
✓ Release the arms and shake them out.
✓ Switch sides and repeat the same steps with the left arm on top and the right arm behind your back.
✓ If you find it hard to reach your hands, don't force it. You can gradually work on improving flexibility in the shoulders over time. Using a strap or towel can be helpful in the beginning to gradually work towards getting the hands closer together.

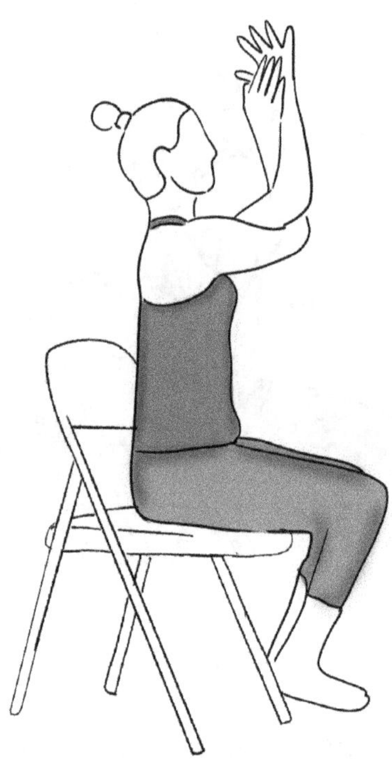

In this case, you should have both your arms extended straight out in front of you at shoulder height. Angle your right arm over your left, bending at the elbows, and bring your palms to touch. If possible, wrap your arms to bring your palms together. Lift your elbows slightly, feeling the stretch between your shoulder blades. Breathe deeply and keep the position for a few little breaths. Unwind the arms and do the same thing with the left arm over the right.

Seated Shoulder Opener

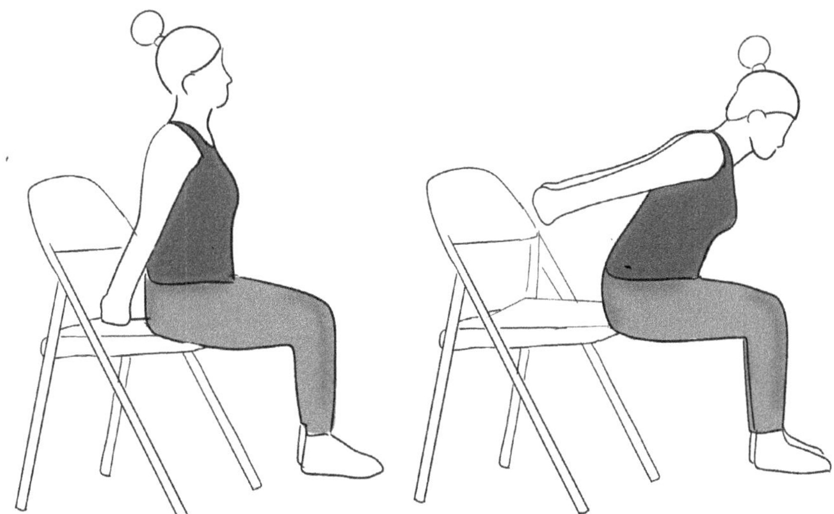

A seated shoulder opener is a gentle yoga stretch that helps to release tension in the shoulders and chest. Let's see how to do it:

- ✓ Sit comfortably on the floor or in a chair with a straight back.
- ✓ Cross your fingers behind your back, with your palms placed inward. If your fingers don't reach, you can use a strap or towel to hold onto, grasping it with both hands.
- ✓ Once your fingers are interlaced, straighten your arms and softly lift them, not close to your body.
- ✓ As you lift your arms, focus on drawing your shoulder blades together and down, opening your chest.
- ✓ Maintain your spine tall and your chest lifted throughout the stretch.
- ✓ Take a few deep breaths as you hold the position, feeling the stretch across your shoulders and chest.
- ✓ If you're comfortable, you can tilt your chin slightly up to enhance the stretch in the front of your chest and throat.
- ✓ Keep in mind not to force the stretch, and only go as far as your body allows. It's essential to always have a sense of relaxation and never strain the muscles.

Seated shoulder openers are particularly helpful if you spend a lot of time sitting at a desk or in front of a computer, as they counteract the rounded shoulders and hunched posture that can develop from these activities. Practicing this stretch regularly can help improve shoulder flexibility and posture.

This stretch will open up the front of your shoulders and chest.

Neck and Shoulder Release

Drop your right ear towards your right shoulder, feeling the stretch along the left side of your neck and shoulder. Keep taking some breaths and moving to the other side.

Seated Neck Circles

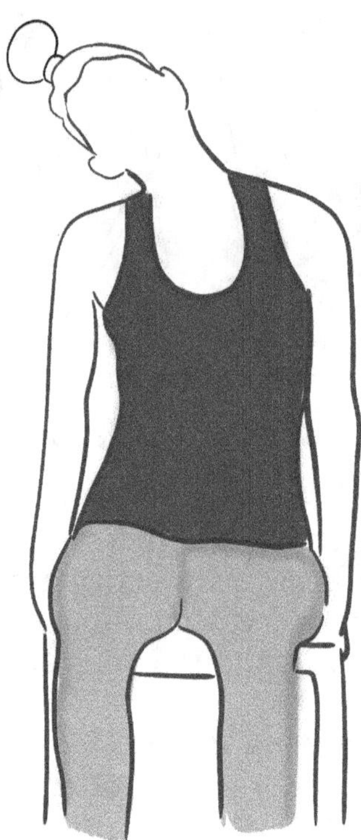

Sit tall and gently roll your neck in a circular motion, moving your head clockwise and then counterclockwise. Be slow and mindful as you do this movement to prevent any strain.

Never forget to breathe deeply and listen to your body during these chair yoga shoulder exercises.

Shoulder yoga, seated, for weight loss

Seated shoulder yoga exercises can be a helpful addition to a comprehensive weight-loss routine. They can improve shoulder mobility and strength, allowing you to engage in more vigorous physical activities and burn calories more effectively. Additionally, yoga helps reduce stress, which may aid in preventing emotional eating and making healthier food choices.

Here's a simple seated shoulder yoga exercise you can try:

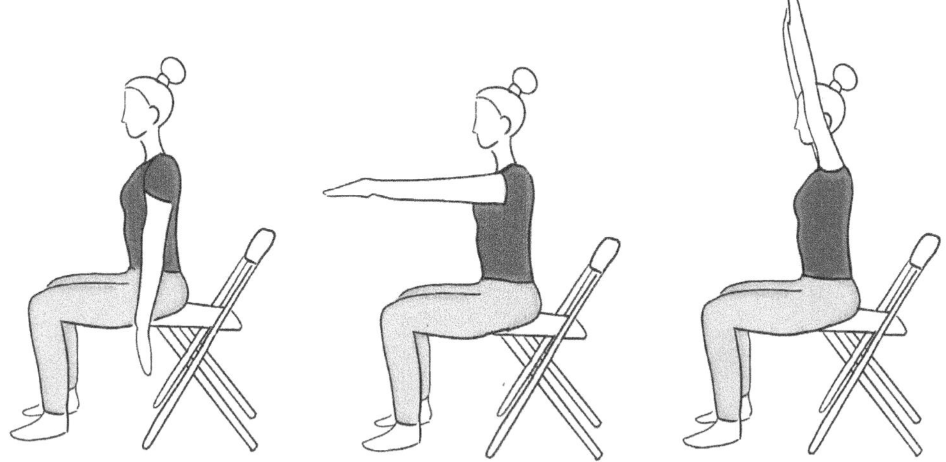

✓ Sit comfortably on a chair. Even in this case, your feet should be placed flat on the floor, and your hands should be on your thighs.
✓ Inhale deeply, and as you exhale, lift both arms up towards the ceiling.
✓ Inhale again, and as you exhale, lower your arms back down to the primary position.
✓ Do this movement for some rounds, matching your breath with the arm raises.
✓ For an added challenge, you can hold light weights or water bottles in each hand while performing the arm raises.

Combining seated shoulder yoga exercises with other forms of exercise, such as cardio and strength training, can help you achieve your weight loss goals more effectively.

Stretch

Let's see a simple chair yoga stretch that you can do to help release tension and promote relaxation:

Seated Forward Bend:

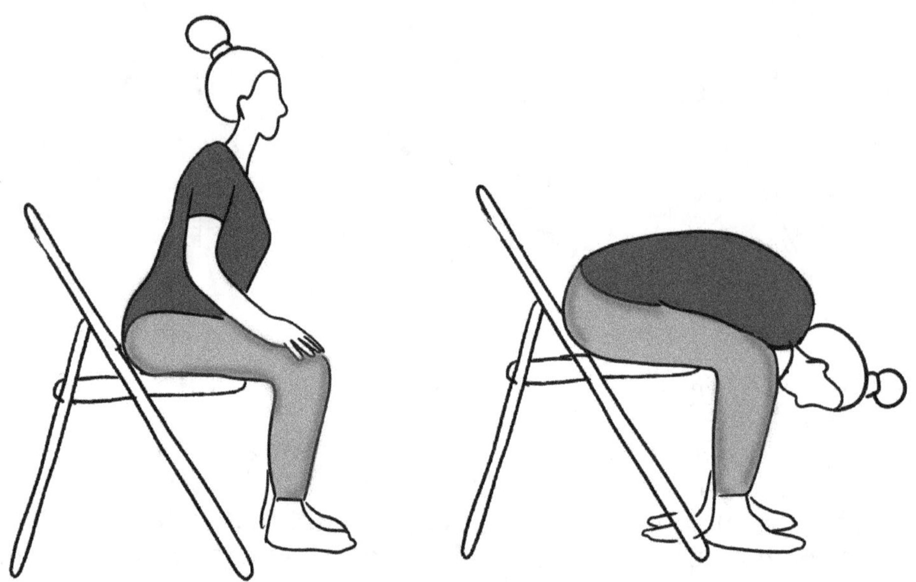

- ✓ One more time, sit comfortably on a chair. The position is the same: your feet flat on the floor and your hands resting on your thighs.
- ✓ Inhale deeply, lengthening your spine, and sit tall.
- ✓ Exhale, and as you do so, hinge at the hips and bend forward, reaching your hands towards your feet or the floor.
- ✓ Let your head and neck relax, allowing your upper body to hang comfortably over your legs.
- ✓ Take a few deep breaths in this position, feeling the stretch along your spine and the back of your legs.
- ✓ Inhale, and as you exhale, slowly sit back up, stacking your vertebrae one on top of the other.
- ✓ Repeat this stretch a few times, focusing on your breath and allowing yourself to release any tension in your body.

This seated forward bend is a gentle stretch that targets the spine, hamstrings, and lower back. It's perfect for easing stiffness and promoting a sense of calm and relaxation. Never forget to move slowly and mindfully, and stay away from any movements that may lead to discomfort or pain.

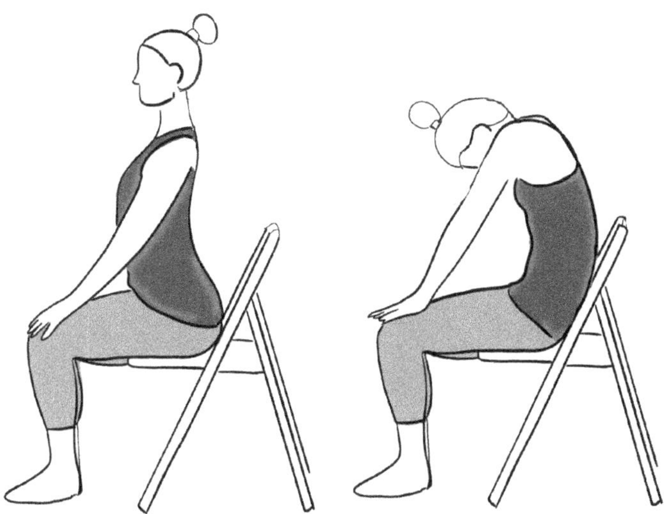

Let's see, in detail now, how to do a proper chair cat-cow stretch:

✓ The same position as sitting on a chair, so feet flat on the floor and hands along your knees.
✓ Inhale deeply as you arch your back and lift your chest, gently gazing upward (Cow pose).
✓ Exhale slowly and round your back, putting your chin towards your chest (Cat pose).
✓ Continue to flow between Cow and Cat poses, matching the movements with your breath.

This seated version of the classic Cat-Cow Stretch helps to mobilize and stretch the spine while seated, promoting flexibility and releasing tension in the back.

Seated Crown Stretch

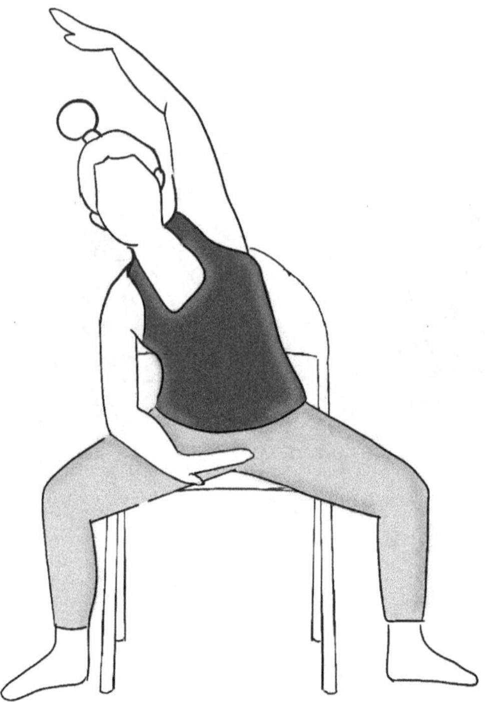

- ✓ Sit comfortably on it like above.
- ✓ Inhale deeply and lengthen your spine, sitting tall.
- ✓ As you exhale, gently drop your head forward, bringing your chin towards your chest.
- ✓ If comfortable, you can use your hands to guide your head slightly deeper into the stretch, feeling a gentle stretch in the back of your neck.
- ✓ Hold this position for a few breaths, then inhale as you slowly lift your head back to an upright position.

The seated crown stretch helps release tension in the neck and upper back, promoting relaxation and reducing stiffness in the neck muscles.

Chair Side Bending and Arm Reach

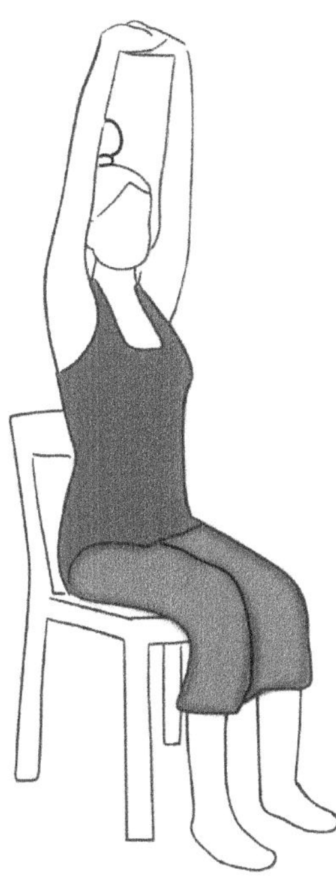

Yoga chair side bending is a yoga pose that involves sitting on a chair with your feet firmly planted on the ground. While holding the backrest of the chair with one hand, you gently stretch your torso sideways, creating a lateral bend along your spine. This helps to increase flexibility, improve posture, and release tension in the sides of the body. It's a variation of traditional side-bending poses that is be executed with the support of a chair.

That's said, let's now see a step-by-step guide on how to perform Yoga chair side bending:

✓ Sit on a sturdy chair with your feet flat on the floor, hip-width apart.
✓ Be certain that your back is straight, and your core is engaged.
✓ Hold the backrest of the chair with your right hand, keeping your elbow slightly bent.
✓ Inhale deeply and lengthen your spine, reaching the crown of your head upward.
✓ As you exhale, gently lean towards the left side, creating a lateral bend along your spine.
✓ Keep your left hand relaxed on your left thigh, or let it hang down toward the floor.
✓ Avoid collapsing your chest or leaning forward; instead, maintain an open chest through-out the movement.
✓ Maintain the stretch and your balance for 20-30 seconds while breathing deeply.
✓ Inhale as you come back to an upright position.
✓ Repeat the same sequence on the other side, holding the chair's backrest with your left hand and bending towards the right.

Even for this pose, perform the movements slowly and mindfully, and never force your body into an uncomfortable position.

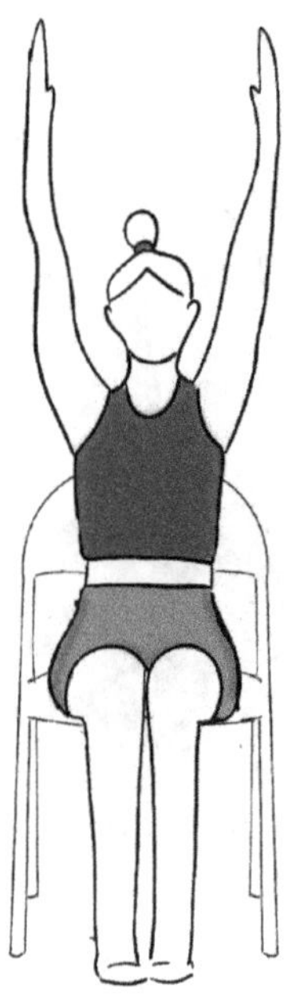

Chair yoga arm reach is a gentle yoga movement performed while seated on a chair. It is an excellent way to improve upper body flexibility and range of motion, making it particularly beneficial for people with mobility or balance challenges. As with any yoga practice, perform the movements mindfully, and avoid overstretching or straining your muscles. If you have any health concerns, consider consulting a yoga instructor or healthcare professional before attempting new exercises.

It involves stretching your arms and upper body to enhance flexibility, release tension, and improve circulation. Let's now see a step-by-step guide on how to perform this pose with the chair:

✓ Sit comfortably on a chair with your feet flat on the floor, hip-width apart, and your spine straight.
✓ Make your shoulders relaxed and place your hands on your thighs.
✓ On an inhale, raise your right arm up toward the ceiling, keeping your palm facing inward.
✓ As you exhale, gently reach your right arm over your head to the left side, creating a gentle stretch along the right side of your body.
✓ Keep your left hand grounded on your chair to maintain stability.
✓ Inhale to come back to an upright position.
✓ Repeat the same movement on the other side, raising your left arm up and stretching it over to the right side.
✓ Continue the flow, alternating sides, for several repetitions, coordinating your breath with the movement.

Chair Pigeon Stretch

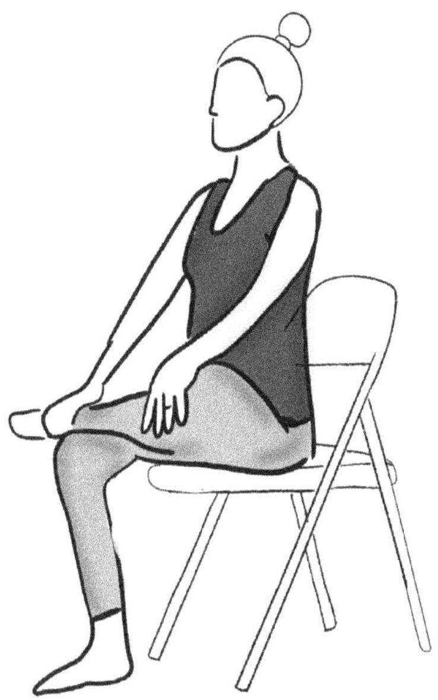

The Chair Pigeon Stretch is a modified version of the Pigeon Pose, a yoga pose that stretch-es and opens up the hips and glutes. It is adapted to be performed while sitting on a chair and is particularly useful for individuals who have difficulty getting down to the floor or have limited mobility. The Chair Pigeon Stretch helps to improve hip flexibility, relieve tension in the hips and lower back, and can be so useful for individuals who spend long periods sitting or have tight hip muscles. As with any yoga or stretching exercise, perform the movement mindfully and avoid pushing yourself too far into the stretch.

Let's see now, how to do the chair pigeon stretch:

✓ Sit comfortably on a chair with your feet flat on the floor, hip-width apart, and your spine straight.
✓ Bring your right ankle to rest on top of your left thigh, just above the knee, forming a figure-four shape with your legs.
✓ Flex your right foot to save your knee and maintain stability.
✓ If you feel a sufficient stretch in this position, stay here and hold the stretch.
✓ For a deeper stretch, lightly lean forward from your hips while keeping your back straight, and this must be done for the moment you will feel a soft stretch in your right hip and glutes.
✓ Keep the stretch for about 20-30 seconds, breathing deeply and relaxing into the stretch.
✓ To release, slowly come back to an upright sitting position and repeat the same stretch on the other side.

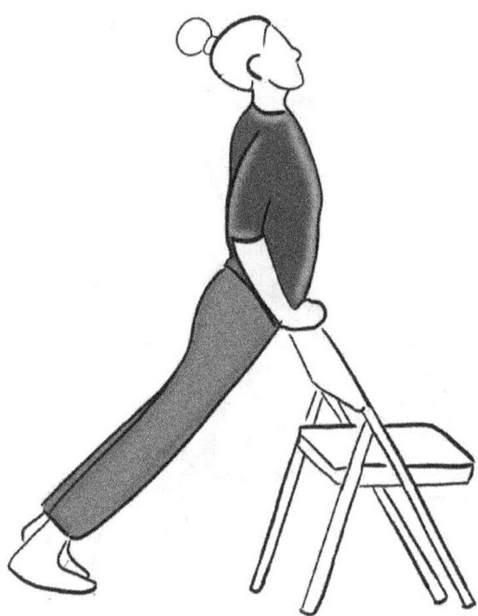

The Cobra Pose Chair is a modified version of the Cobra Pose, a back bend yoga pose that stretches the chest, shoulders, and abdomen while strengthening the spine and improving posture.

The Cobra Pose Chair variation provides similar benefits to the traditional Cobra Pose, such as improving back strength, stretching the front body, and enhancing overall flexibility. It is an excellent option for those who want to incorporate back bends into their practice while using the stability of a chair for support. As with any yoga pose, practice with awareness and listen to your body, making adjustments as needed to ensure a safe and comfortable experience

The chair variation is adapted to be performed with the support of a chair, making it accessible for individuals who may have difficulty getting down to the floor or need additional support. Here's the definition of the Cobra Pose Chair:

✓ Again, place yourself in a chair with your feet flat on the floor. You must also place your hip-width apart, and your hands on your thighs.
✓ Slide your hands down the sides of the chair and place them on the seat, slightly behind your hips, with your fingers pointing forward.
✓ Maintain your elbows next to your body and your shoulders relaxed.
✓ Inhale deeply and press your palms into the chair seat while gently arching your back and lifting your chest forward and upward.
✓ Maintain a slight engagement of your core muscles and lengthen your spine during the movement.
✓ Keep the pose for 15-30 seconds, breathing deeply and allowing your chest to open and expand.
✓ Exhale as you slowly release the pose and sit upright again.

Chair yoga pose variants, as we have seen so far, are excellent for promoting flexibility, strength, and relaxation. Some popular variants include seated twists, forward bends, and gentle back bends. It's always important to focus on your breath and listen to your body while doing these poses. Always consult a qualified yoga instructor for proper guidance. In the next chapter, your chair yoga journey goes on!

CHAPTER 6

CHAIR YOGA AND MUSCLE TONING FOCUS

In the previous chapter, our attention was mainly directed to the variations of the classic yoga poses, in this one, we will concentrate on muscle tone. Here you will find fantastic, simple, and quick exercises to always do in the chair that will help you tone up and clean up your muscles!

Chair yoga and muscle toning

In chair yoga, you can target various muscle groups for toning and strengthening. Some key areas to focus on include the core muscles, such as the abdominals and obliques, by incorporating seated twists and side bends. You can engage the leg muscles with chair squats and leg lifts. For upper body toning, try incorporating seated arm exercises like bicep curls, triceps extensions, and shoulder presses. But it's essential to maintain proper form and practice regularly to see improvements in muscle tone and overall strength.

Chair yoga can be an effective way to tone and strengthen muscles, especially for individuals with limited mobility or physical limitations. By using the support of a chair, you can do a number of exercises that are focused on different muscle groups. Chair yoga poses often require you to engage your core, arms, legs, and back, which helps to tone these areas.

Additionally, chair yoga promotes body awareness and mindfulness, encouraging you to focus on your breath and muscle engagement during the practice. Consistent practice of chair yoga can lead to improved muscle tone, flexibility, and overall strength.

However, it's important to note that while chair yoga can be beneficial, it may not provide the same level of muscle toning as more vigorous forms of exercise. It is best suited for individuals seeking a gentle and accessible way to improve muscle strength and flexibility, especially those with lower mobility or physical issues. As with any fitness routine, combining chair yoga with other forms of exercise can provide a well-rounded approach to achieving your fitness goals.

A general overview: best chair yoga positions for a better muscle tone

Let's see a general overview to guide you on the best positions of chair yoga to perform for a better muscle tone. Let's start with the glutes. Before starting, keep in mind that consistent practice will help tone and strengthen your glutes over time.

GLUTES

Chair yoga can be a functional way to tone your glutes. Let's see some chair yoga poses that can help:

- ✓ Chair Pigeon Pose: Sit on the edge of a chair with one ankle crossed over the opposite knee. Incline forward slightly to perceive the stretch in your glutes.
- ✓ Chair Warrior II Pose: Sit with your legs wide apart and turn one foot out. At the same time, you should keep your other foot forward. Bend the knee of the turned-out foot and extend the other leg. This pose engages the glutes.
- ✓ Chair Bridge Pose: Sit on the chair, and in this case, your feet must be flat on the ground, hip-width apart. Press through your feet and lift your hips up, squeezing your glutes as you do so.
- ✓ Chair Squats: Stand in front of the chair with your feet shoulder-width apart. Lower yourself into a sitting position, almost touching the chair, then stand back up, engaging your glutes throughout the movement.

LEGS

Chair yoga can indeed help tone your legs. So, we want to show you now some chair yoga poses that target your leg muscles:

✓ Chair Forward Fold: Sit on the chair with your feet flat on the ground. This stretches and engages the hamstrings and calves.
✓ Chair High Lunge: Sit on the edge of the chair, extend one leg straight back, and rest the ball of your foot on the ground. Hold the other knee at a 90-degree angle, creating a lunge position. This pose works your quadriceps and glutes.
✓ Chair Tree Pose: Sit with your feet flat on the ground. Lift one foot off the floor and put the sole against the inner thigh of the opposite leg. Engage your standing leg for balance and strength.
✓ Chair Warrior III Pose: Sit on the chair and hinge forward from the hips, extending one leg straight back while keeping your body parallel to the ground. This pose targets your hamstrings and challenges your balance.
✓ Chair Calf Raises: in this case, you must place yourself on the chair, always with your feet flat on the ground. Lift your heels off the floor to come up into your toes, then lower them back down. This exercise targets your calf muscles.

As a final tip, it's essential to breathe deeply and focus on proper alignment in each pose. Regular practice of these chair yoga poses is always essential if your aim is to tone and strengthen your leg muscles over time.

ABDOMINAL

Chair yoga can be beneficial for toning your abdominal muscles. So, see again some chair yoga poses that target the core:

✓ Seated Cat-Cow Stretch: Sit on the chair with your feet flat on the ground. Put your hands on your knees. Inhale and arch your back, lifting your chest and looking up (Cow Pose). Do the cat pose and repeat this gentle movement to engage your core.
✓ Seated Spinal Twist: Sit on the chair in the same way. Twist your torso to one side, holding the back of the chair for support. This pose targets the obliques and helps improve spinal mobility.
✓ Seated Boat Pose: Sit on the edge of the chair, lean slightly back, and lift your legs off the ground, keeping them bent. Balancing on your sit bones, expand your arms forward. This pose engages your core muscles.
✓ Seated Knee Tucks: Sit the same way. Lift one knee toward your chest, engaging your abdominal muscles. Lower the foot back down and switch to the other leg. Repeat alternately.
✓ Seated Belly Breathing: Sit comfortably on the chair with your hands positioned on your belly. Inhale deeply, expanding your belly, and exhale fully, drawing your navel towards your spine. This breathing exercise activates and strengthens your deep abdominal muscles.

Never forget to maintain proper alignment and perform the movements mindfully. Consistent practice of these chair yoga poses can be useful to strengthen and tone your abdominal muscles, at the same time your abdominal muscles during the practice.

Chair Leg Extension

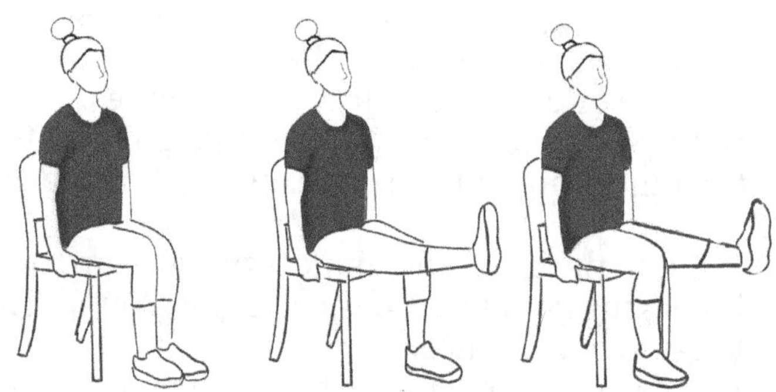

Chair leg extension, in the context of exercise or fitness, refers to a movement that involves extending one leg while seated on a chair or a similar stable surface. It is a strengthening exercise that first focuses on the quadriceps muscles, which are located in the front of the thigh. The movement is typically performed by sitting upright on the chair, with the feet flat on the floor. Then, one leg is straightened and lifted off the ground, extending it fully or partially while keeping the knee aligned and stable. The leg is then lowered back to the starting position.

Chair leg extensions are often used in rehabilitation settings or as a part of a seated exercise routine for individuals with limited mobility or those who need a low-impact option for strengthening the leg muscles. This exercise can be modified based on the individual's abilities and fitness level, making it accessible to a wide range of people. As with any exercise, it's vital to do chair leg extensions with appropriate form and control to prevent injury and achieve the desired benefits.

Anyway, to perform chair leg extensions, follow these steps:

✓ Sit upright on a sturdy chair with your back straight and feet flat on the floor, hip-width apart.
✓ Put your hands on the sides of the chair or grip the seat for balance and stability.
✓ Choose one leg to start with. Slowly extend that leg forward, straightening it as much as you can comfortably manage. Keep your knee aligned and avoid locking it.
✓ Hold the extended position briefly, engaging your quadriceps (front thigh muscles).
✓ Lower your extended leg back down to the beginning position with control.
✓ Repeat the movement for the same leg, aiming for 10-15 repetitions.
✓ Move on to the other leg and perform the same number of repetitions.

TIPS:

✓ Keep your core engaged throughout the exercise for better stability and support.
✓ Focus on controlled movements, avoiding jerky motions.
✓ You can increase or decrease the difficulty of the exercise by adjusting the range of motion or adding ankle weights if you're looking for more challenge.

And finally, it's vital to keep in mind that you should perform these exercises within your own comfort and ability levels.

Chair Leg Curl

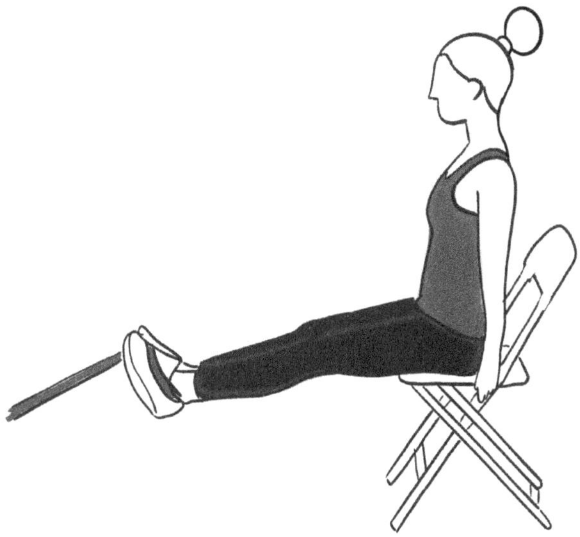

The chair leg curl is a lower-body exercise that targets the hamstring muscles, which are placed at the back of your thighs. It is a variation of the traditional leg curl exercise commonly performed on a specialized machine at the gym.

To perform the chair leg curl, you sit on a chair with your feet flat on the floor. Then, you extend your legs out in front of you and slowly bend your knees to curl your legs back towards your body, focusing on contracting your hamstring muscles. Hold the curled position for a moment, and then lower your legs back down to the starting position.

This exercise can be an effective way to strengthen and tone your hamstrings, which play an essential role in various daily activities, as well as sports and fitness routines. The chair leg curl is a simple yet beneficial exercise that can be done at home or in the office using a sturdy chair. Always keep proper form and control throughout the movement to maximize its success and minimize the risk of injury. Let's see some variants.

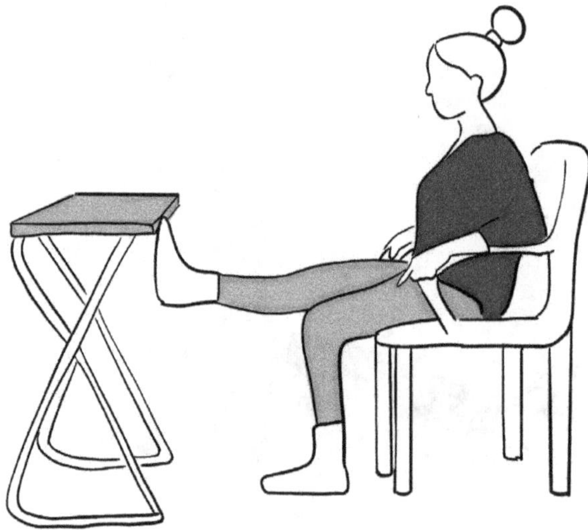

Sit on a chair with your feet flat on the floor. Extend your legs out in front of you and then slowly bend your knees to curl your legs back towards your body, engaging your hamstring muscles. Hold for a moment and then lower your legs back down.

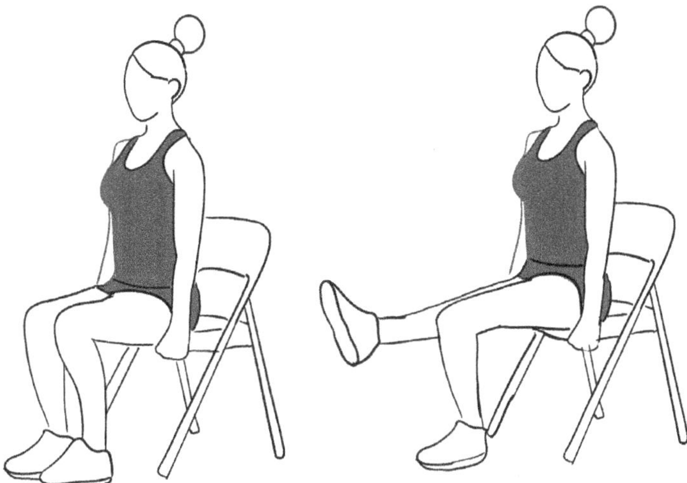

Sit on the edge of a chair with one leg extended straight out in front of you and the other foot flat on the floor. Bend the extended leg at the knee to curl it back towards your body, engaging the hamstring. Maintain for a moment and then lower it back down. Do the same on the other leg.

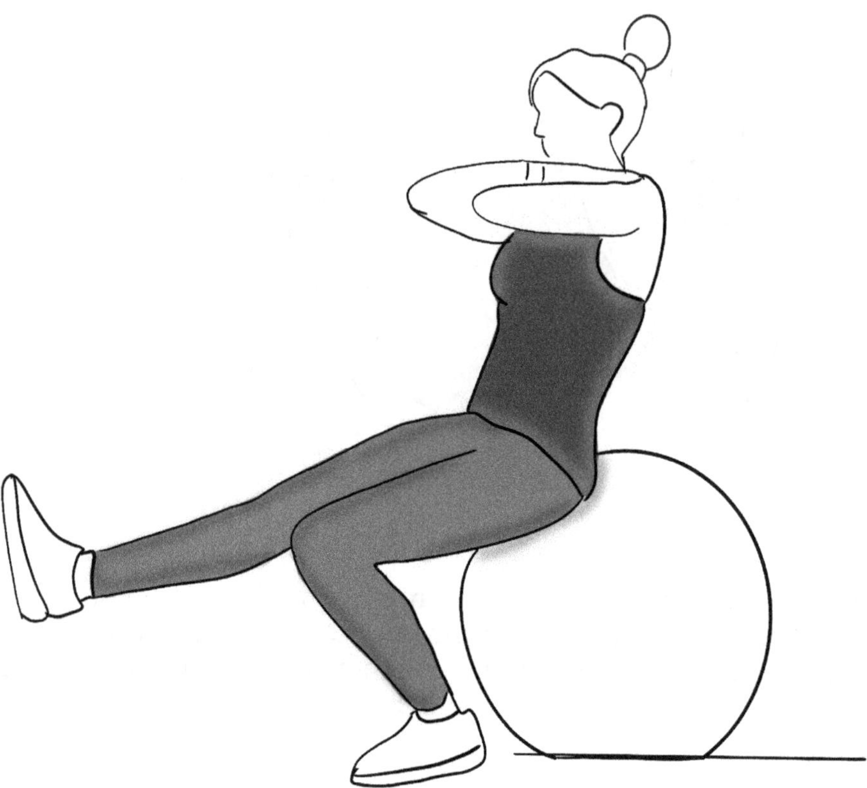

Place a Swiss ball in front of a chair. Lie on your back with your heels resting on top of the ball. Lift your hips off the floor and use your heels to roll the ball towards your body, bending your knees. Put your legs expanded back out and do again the movement.

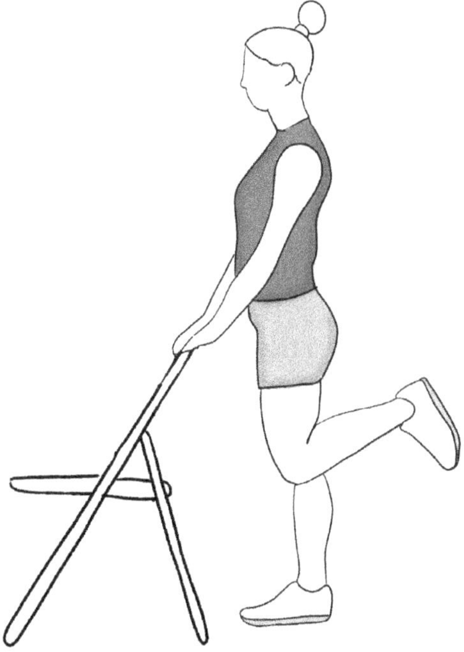

Stand facing the back of a chair, holding onto the top for support. Bend one knee behind you and curl your heel up towards your glutes, engaging your hamstring. Lower your leg back down and do the same on the other leg.

Chair Standing Up

The term "chair standing up" typically refers to the action of transitioning from a seated position to a standing position while using a chair for support or assistance. This movement is a common daily activity that most people perform numerous times throughout the day.

When someone mentions "chair standing up," they are likely referring to the process of sitting on a chair and then using their leg muscles and core strength to lift themselves off the chair and stand upright. This action involves pushing through the feet, straightening the hips and knees, and engaging the muscles necessary for maintaining balance and stability.

The skill of standing up from a chair is a fundamental movement that impacts one's functional independence and overall mobility. People who have difficulties with this action may benefit from exercises to strengthen their leg muscles, core, and overall stability to enhance their ability to perform this activity with ease and confidence. Additionally, individuals with specific mobility challenges may use adaptive devices or support systems to assist them in standing up.

However, we want to show you a step-by-step guide:

- ✓ Sit at the edge of the chair with your feet flat on the floor, shoulder-width apart.
- ✓ Put your hands on the armrests or on the seat beside your thighs for support.
- ✓ Lean forward slightly and activate your core muscles.
- ✓ Push through your heels and use your leg muscles to lift your body off the chair.
- ✓ Straighten your hips and stand tall.
- ✓ Maintain good posture by keeping your back straight and your shoulders relaxed.
- ✓ Once standing, pause for a moment to ensure your balance.
- ✓ When you're ready to sit back down, reverse the steps by bending your knees, shifting your hips back, and lowering yourself onto the chair in a controlled manner.

It's essential to take your time and avoid rushing the process, especially if you have any mobility or balance issues. If you find it challenging to stand up from a chair, consider using armrests or a sturdy support to assist you. Additionally, regular exercise and strength training can be useful in improving your skills to execute everyday activities like standing up from a chair with ease.

Chair Box Squat

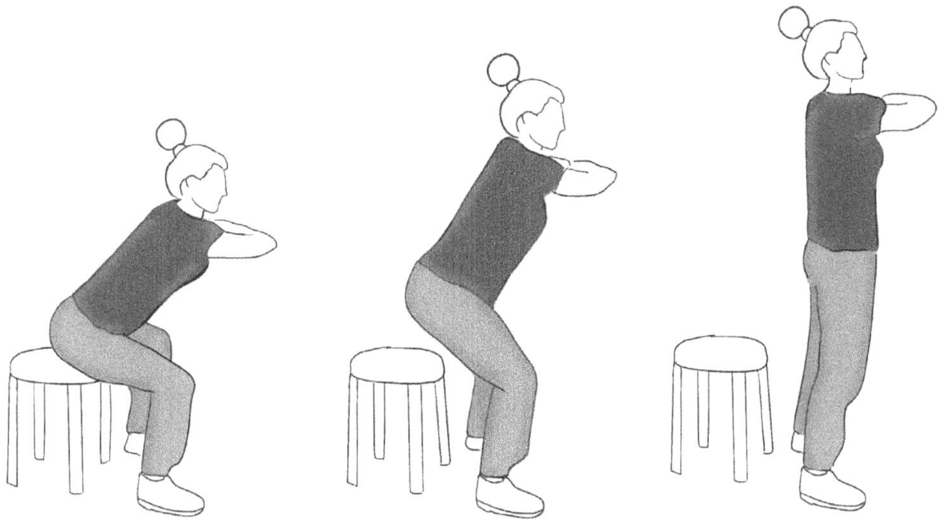

The chair box squat is a variation of the traditional squat exercise that involves using a chair or box as a reference point to control the depth and form of the movement. We are talking about a truly useful exercise for enhancing lower body strength, especially in the quadriceps, hamstrings, and gluteal muscles, while improving overall squatting mechanics as well.

The chair box squat is an excellent exercise for those who are new to squatting or have limited mobility, as it provides a reference point to gauge depth and maintain proper form.

Let's see how to perform a chair box squat:

✓ Position a sturdy chair or a box behind you, ensuring it is stable and won't move during the exercise.
✓ Place yourself with your feet shoulder-width apart and your toes slightly turned out.
✓ Also, activate your core and keep your chest lifted throughout the movement.
✓ Begin the squat by pushing your hips back and bending your knees, as if you were about to sit on the chair or box behind you.
✓ Lower yourself down in a controlled manner, ensuring your knees stay in line with your toes and your back remains straight.
✓ Have the purpose to lower yourself until your glutes gently touch the chair or box, or until your thighs are parallel to the ground. You can change and regulate the depth depending on your comfort and flexibility.
✓ Pause briefly at the bottom position, maintaining tension in your muscles.
✓ Push through your heels, engage your leg muscles, and stand back up to the starting position.

Chair Calf Raises

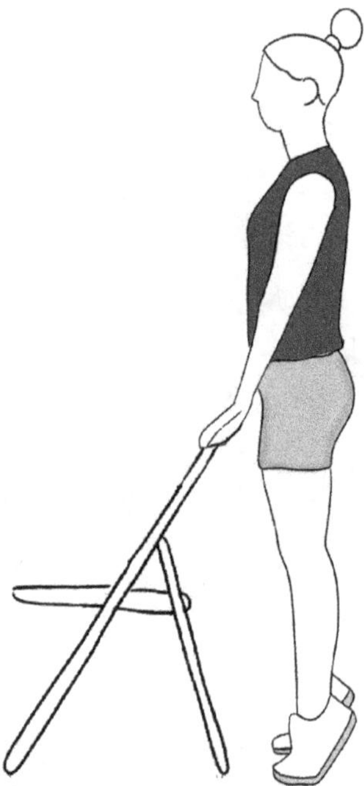

Chair calf raises are a calf-strengthening exercise that can be performed while sitting on a chair. They target the muscles in the calves, specifically the gastrocnemius and soles muscles, which are located in the back of your lower legs. This exercise is easy and can be executed almost anywhere with a sturdy chair.

Here's how to do chair calf raises:

✓ Sit on a chair with your feet flat on the floor, hip-width apart.
✓ Put your hands on your thighs or the sides of the chair for a more balance.
✓ Keeping your heels on the floor, lift your toes and the balls of your feet as high as possible.
✓ Keep the raised position for a moment, and you should also perceive the contraction in your calf area.
✓ Lower your heels back down slowly to return to the first position.
✓ Do these calf raises for several repetitions, aiming for 10-15 reps or as many as you can comfortably perform.

As you become more proficient, you can improve the difficulty by holding weights on your thighs or using one leg at a time. Calf raises help improve calf strength and stability, and can be beneficial for activities that involve walking, running, or jumping.

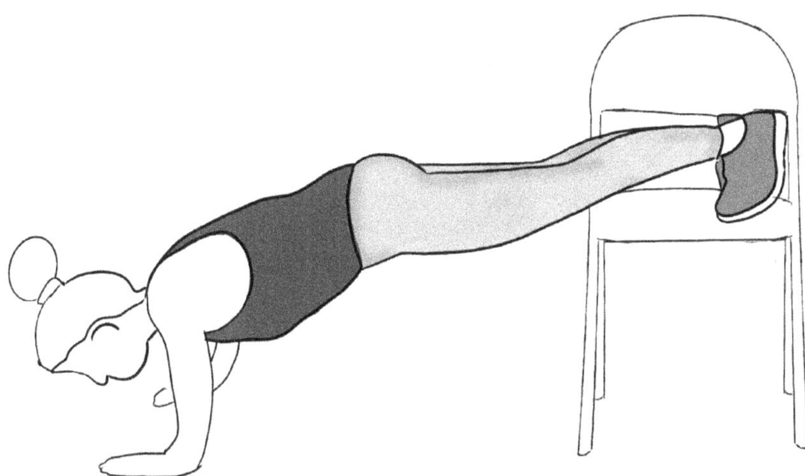

It refers to a push-up variation that involves using a chair for support or elevation to modify the traditional push-up exercise. In this variation, you might place your hands on the seat of a chair while positioning your body at an incline to reduce the resistance and intensity of the push-up.

If this is indeed the exercise you are referring to, here's how you could perform a chair leg push-up:

✓ Place a sturdy chair with a stable base in front of you.
✓ Have a push-up position with your hands on the seat of the chair and your arms straight.
✓ Walk your feet back to create a diagonal line from your head to your heels.
✓ Engage your core, maintain your body straight, and lower your chest towards the chair by bending your elbows.
✓ Push through your hands to straighten your arms and return to the starting position.

Chair Arm Circles

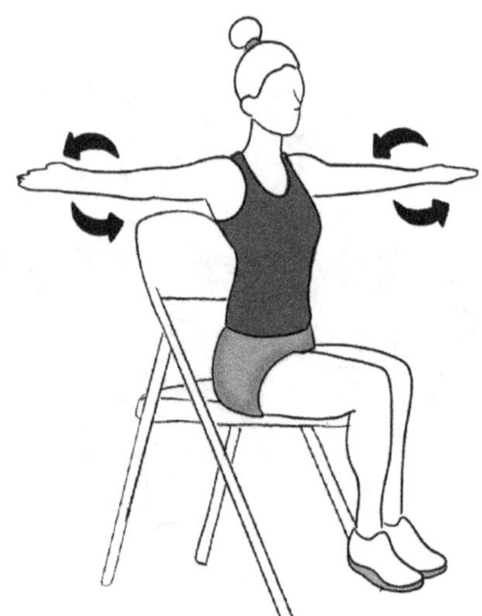

Chair arm circles are a form of exercise where you sit on a chair with your feet flat on the floor and your back straight. Then, you extend your arms out to the sides and perform a circular motions with your arms. This exercise is functional for improving shoulder mobility and flexibility.

To perform chair arm circles, follow these steps:

✓ Sit on a chair with your back straight, but you should also have your feet well flat on the floor.
✓ Expand your arms out to the sides at shoulder height.
✓ Keep your palms facing down or forward, whichever is more comfortable.
✓ Begin making circular motions with your arms. Begin with small circles and lower, the size if you can do so comfortably.
✓ Do the circles again for a set number of repetitions or time (e.g., 10 circles clockwise, then 10 circles counterclockwise).
✓ Focus on keeping your movements controlled and steady during the exercise performance.
✓ You can incorporate chair arm circles into your warm-up routine or employ them as a fast break from sitting for extended periods.

As a final tip, it's always a good idea to listen to your body and stop immediately if you experience any discomfort or pain.

Chair Lifted Hip

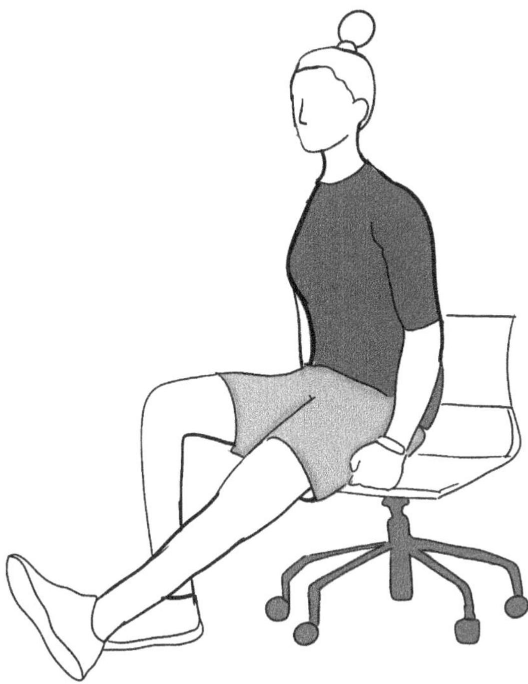

In chair yoga, the term "lifted hip" refers to an exercise or pose that involves raising one hip higher than the other while sitting on a chair. This movement is typically done to stretch and engage the hip muscles, improve flexibility, and promote balance and stability.

To do the lifted hip exercise in chair yoga:

- ✓ Sit on a chair, always with your back straight and your feet well-placed on the ground.
- ✓ So, put your hands on the sides of the chair for major support and balance.
- ✓ Lift one hip off the chair slightly, creating a tilt in your pelvis to that side.
- ✓ Keep the other hip grounded on the chair and maintain an even distribution of weight on both feet.
- ✓ Maintain the lifted hip position for a few breaths, feeling the stretch in the side of your body.
- ✓ Decrease the lifted hip back to the chair and repeat on the other side.

This exercise can be beneficial for those with limited mobility or who may find it challenging to perform traditional standing or floor-based yoga poses. It can be useful when it comes to opening up the hips, improving core strength, and improving body awareness. As with any exercise, it's essential to perform it with control and within your comfort range to avoid strain or injury.

Chair Shuffle Leg

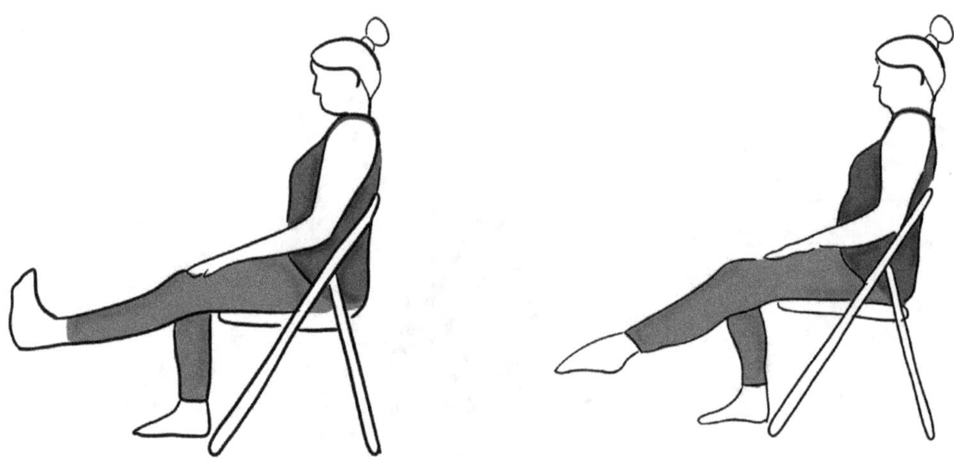

In the context of fitness or exercise, the "chair shuffle leg" likely refers to a movement or exercise performed while sitting on a chair to engage and strengthen the leg muscles.

To perform the chair shuffle leg exercise:

✓ Sit on a chair with your back straight and your feet flat on the floor.
✓ Put your hands one more time on the sides of the chair for support.
✓ Lift one foot slightly off the ground while keeping the other foot firmly planted.
✓ Shuffle the lifted foot forward and backward, or side to side, as if you were sliding it on the floor while remaining seated.
✓ Execute the movement for some number of repetitions or a specific duration.
✓ Move on to the other leg and do the exercise again.

The chair shuffle leg exercise can be a simple and effective way to work on leg strength, stability, and mobility, especially for those who have difficulty standing or performing weight-bearing exercises. It can also be used as a gentle warm-up or as part of a seated workout routine. As always, listen to your body, and if you experience any discomfort or pain, stop the exercise immediately.

Toe Taps and Arm Reach

Chair yoga toe taps and arm reach are two separate exercises that can be performed while sitting on a chair to promote flexibility and mobility.

Chair Yoga Toe Taps:

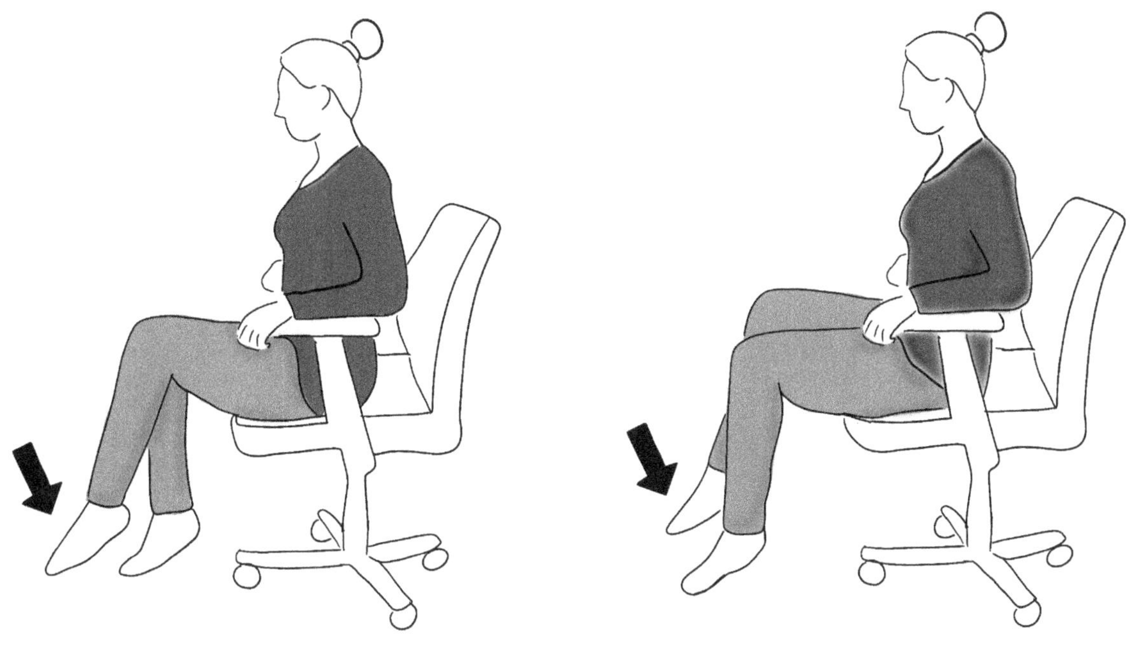

✓ Sit on a chair again with your feet well flat on the ground.
✓ Lift one foot off the floor, expanding your leg forward.
✓ Gently tap the toes of the lifted foot on the floor while keeping the rest of your body still.
✓ Lift the foot back up, and then switch to the other leg.
✓ Repeat the toe taps on each leg for some repetitions.

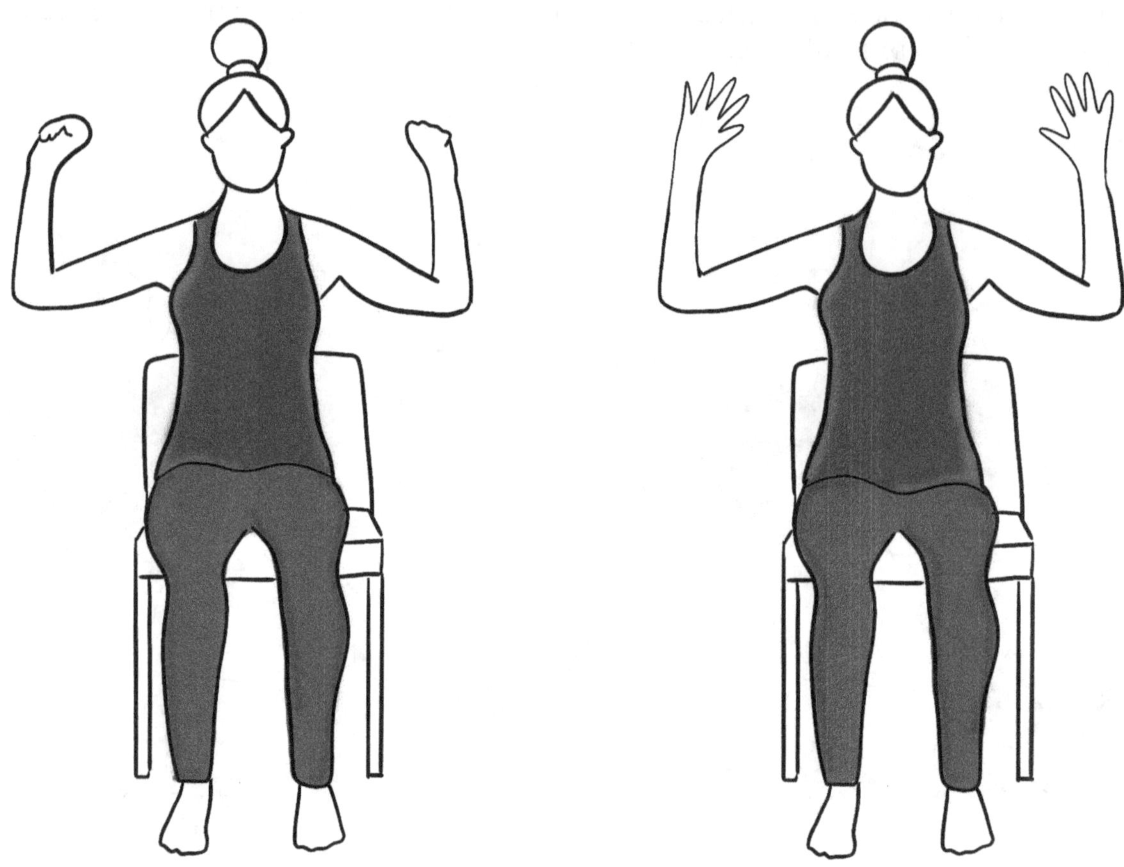

- ✓ Sit on a chair. Again, keep your back straight and your feet flat.
- ✓ Put your arms out in front of you, well extended and at shoulder height.
- ✓ Inhale deeply, and as you exhale, reach your arms forward as if you are trying to touch something in front of you.
- ✓ Inhale one more time and put your arms back in the first position.
- ✓ Repeat the arm reach movement for some repetitions or other times.

Both of these chair yoga exercises can be beneficial for increasing circulation, improving joint flexibility, and enhancing overall body awareness. They are gentle and suitable for individuals with mobility challenges or those who prefer a seated workout. Always perform these exercises at your own pace and within your comfort level.

Final thoughts on chair yoga and muscle-toning exercises

Chair yoga and muscle-toning exercises are excellent options for individuals who may have limited mobility, prefer a seated workout, or are looking for gentle exercises to improve strength and flexibility. Before concluding this chapter, we want to give you some final thoughts on these two types of exercises:

Chair Yoga:

Chair yoga gives a soft and accessible approach to yoga, making it suitable for people of all fitness levels and ages.

It helps improve flexibility, balance, and posture while promoting relaxation and reducing stress.

Chair yoga is beneficial for individuals with mobility issues, seniors, office workers, or anyone who spends long hours sitting.

Regular practice of chair yoga can enhance body awareness and mindfulness.

Muscle-Toning Exercises:

Muscle-toning exercises focus on strengthening and sculpting specific muscle groups in the body.

They can be done with body weight, resistance bands, or light weights to challenge the muscles effectively.

These exercises help improve muscle definition, metabolism, and overall physical performance.

Muscle-toning workouts can be suitable for different fitness levels, making them suitable for beginners and advanced exercisers.

Combining chair yoga and muscle-toning exercises can create a well-rounded fitness routine that addresses both flexibility and strength. It's always the best idea to listen to your body, begin at a comfortable level, and progress gradually to avoid injury.

To end, it's always essential to keep in mind that staying consistent with exercise and choosing activities you enjoy are key factors in maintaining a healthy and active lifestyle.

CHAPTER 7

CHAIR YOGA AND CARDIO FOCUS

If in the last chapter we talked about chair yoga and muscle tone, now we will concentrate better on cardio, or rather, the activity that helps us burn more calories and therefore lose weight faster. We will see the relationship between cardio and chair yoga, and which exercises to perform to achieve our goal. Let's begin!

Relation between chair yoga and cardio

Chair yoga and cardio are two different types of physical activities that can offer unique benefits for overall health and well-being.

Chair yoga, as we have seen many times, focuses on gentle stretching, breathing exercises, and relaxation techniques. It is especially beneficial for individuals with limited mobility or physical restrictions, as it reduces the need to get down on the floor.

Cardio, short for cardiovascular exercise, refers to activities that expand your heart rate and breathing. For some examples of cardio, we have running, cycling, or jumping rope. These exercises are great for improving cardiovascular fitness, stamina, and burning calories.

While chair yoga may not provide the same level of intensity as traditional cardio exercises, it still offers numerous health benefits, including improved flexibility, better posture, reduced stress, and increased mindfulness. Incorporating chair yoga into a sedentary lifestyle can be a great way to start moving and enjoy the benefits of physical activity, especially for those who find traditional cardio exercises challenging.

For a well-rounded fitness routine, combining chair yoga with regular cardio exercises can be beneficial. Cardiovascular activities help to improve cardiovascular health and stamina, while chair yoga complements them by focusing on flexibility, relaxation, and gentle movement. The combination can provide a balanced approach to fitness, catering to different needs and fitness levels. As always, it's essential to ask a healthcare professional before starting any new exercise regimen, especially if you have any pre-existing health conditions.

Chair yoga and cardio focus

Chair yoga primarily focuses on promoting mindfulness, reducing stress, and increasing mobility, making it a suitable option for people with limited mobility or physical challenges.

Cardiovascular exercises, on the other hand, primarily focus on improving cardiovascular fitness. The main goal is to elevate your heart rate and breathing, which helps strengthen the heart, improve lung capacity, and burn calories. Activities like running, cycling, dancing, and jumping rope are common examples of cardio workouts.

While chair yoga may not have the same intense cardiovascular focus as traditional cardio exercises, it still offers significant benefits for overall well-being. Combining chair yoga with regular cardio workouts can create a well-rounded fitness routine that addresses flexibility, strength, balance, relaxation, and cardiovascular health.

The match between chair yoga and cardio depends on individual preferences, fitness goals, and physical abilities. Some people may prefer chair yoga for its gentle approach and mind-body connection, while others may opt for cardio exercises to improve endurance and burn calories. For a comprehensive fitness routine, incorporating elements of both chair yoga and cardio can provide a balanced and holistic approach to health and fitness, but above all, for better weight loss.

Seated March

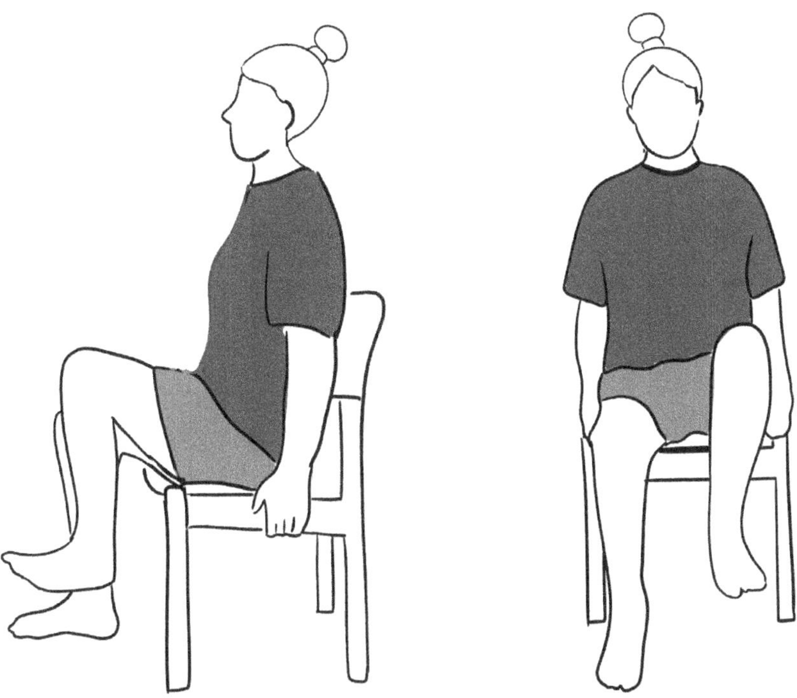

Seated March is an exercise that is typically performed in a seated position, often on a chair or stability ball. It involves lifting and lowering each leg alternately, mimicking the motion of marching while sitting down. Seated marches are a low-impact exercise that can be suitable for people with limited mobility, those recovering from injuries, or individuals who prefer seated exercises. This movement helps in engaging the leg muscles, increasing circulation, and promoting joint mobility. It can be a part of a gentle exercise routine, a warm-up before more intense workouts, or used during a sedentary period to add some physical activity.

To execute a seated march:

✓ Sit up straight with your feet flat on the floor, hip-width apart.
✓ Put your hands on the sides of the chair or hold onto the edges of the seat for support.
✓ Lift one knee towards your chest, while maintaining the other foot on the floor.
✓ Lower the lifted leg back down to the first position.
✓ Do the motion with the other leg, alternating between legs in a controlled and rhythmic manner.

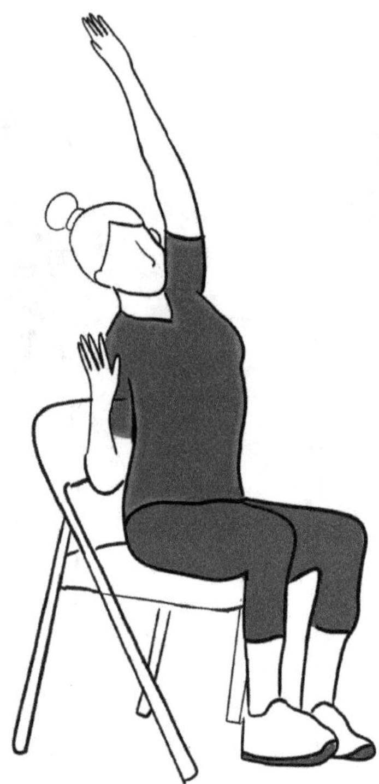

The seated march with opposite arm reach is a variation of the traditional seated march exercise that incorporates additional upper body movement. In addition to lifting and lowering each leg alternately, you also reach the opposite arm overhead, adding a stretching component to the exercise. This exercise combines the benefits of the seated march (engaging the leg muscles, increasing circulation, and promoting joint mobility) with an added upper body stretch, helping to improve flexibility and range of motion in the shoulders and arms. It can be an excellent option for a full-body seated workout, especially for individuals looking to incorporate both leg and upper body movements while seated, such as seniors or individuals with mobility challenges. To perform a seated march with opposite arm reach:

✓ Sit up straight with your feet flat on the ground, hip-width apart.
✓ Put your hands on the sides of the chair or hold onto the edges of the seat for support.
✓ Lift one knee towards your chest, while simultaneously reaching the opposite arm overhead towards the ceiling.
✓ Decrease the lifted leg and arm back down to the beginning position.
✓ Repeat the motion with the other leg and opposite arm, alternating between legs and arms in a controlled and rhythmic manner.

Chair Rotation

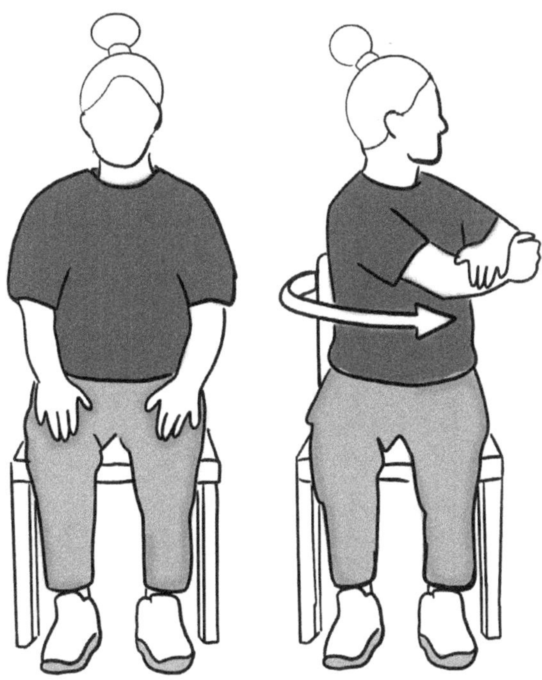

Cardio chair rotation is a seated exercise that combines cardiovascular movement with core engagement. It involves rotating the upper body from side to side while sitting on a chair, providing a low-impact way to get the heart rate up and work the abdominal and oblique muscles.

To perform cardio chair rotation:

✓ Sit upright on a chair with your feet flat on the floor, hip-width apart.
✓ Hold your hands together in front of your chest or place them behind your head for added support.
✓ Activate your core muscles by pulling your belly button towards your spine.
✓ Start rotating your upper body to the right side, twisting from the waist while keeping your hips stable.
✓ Return to the center and then rotate your upper body to the left side, again twisting from the waist.
✓ Continue this side-to-side rotation in a controlled and rhythmic manner.
✓ As you perform cardio chair rotation, focus on the movement coming from your torso, not just your arms. Breathe steadily throughout the exercise and maintain good posture to protect your back.

This seated exercise is an excellent option for individuals who may have difficulty with standing or high-impact cardio workouts. It helps increase blood flow, burn calories, and engage the core muscles, which can contribute to improved stability and balance.

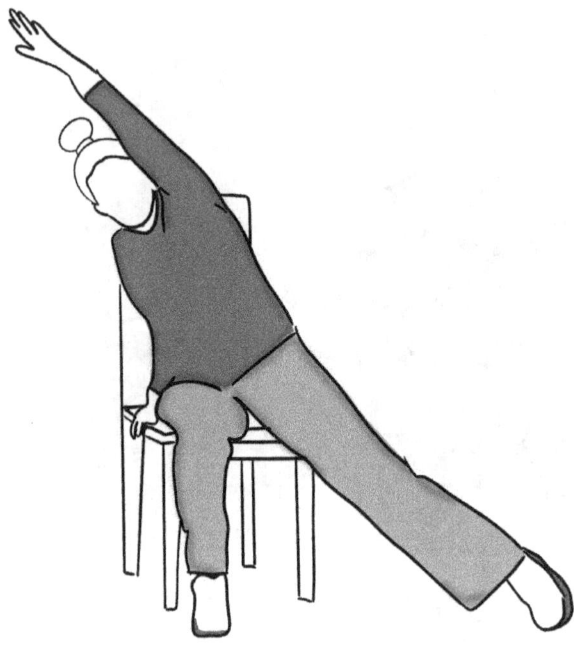

Cardio Chair Yoga Step and Reach is a dynamic seated exercise that combines elements of cardio, yoga, and stretching. It involves rhythmic movements of stepping and reaching while sitting on a chair, promoting cardiovascular fitness, flexibility, and overall body movement. The combination of stepping and reaching movements engages the leg muscles, promotes circulation, and elevates the heart rate, providing a cardio aspect to the exercise. Additionally, the reaching motion helps to stretch the upper body, shoulders, and arms, while also improving flexibility and coordination.

To perform cardio chair yoga step and reach:

✓ Sit comfortably on a chair with your feet flat on the floor, hip-width apart.
✓ Hold your hands together in front of your chest or rest them on your thighs.
✓ Start by lifting your right foot off the floor and stepping it slightly forward, as if taking a step.
✓ At the same time, reach both arms overhead and slightly forward, stretching upward.
✓ Put your right foot back to the beginning position and lower your arms back to the initial position.
✓ Now, lift your left foot off the floor and repeat the same step and reach movement on the opposite side.
✓ Continue alternating between the right and left sides in a fluid and controlled manner.

Cardio Chair Yoga Step and Reach can be a suitable option for people with limited mobility or those who prefer seated exercises. It offers a gentle yet effective way to get the body moving and increase the heart rate without putting stress on the joints.

Assisted March

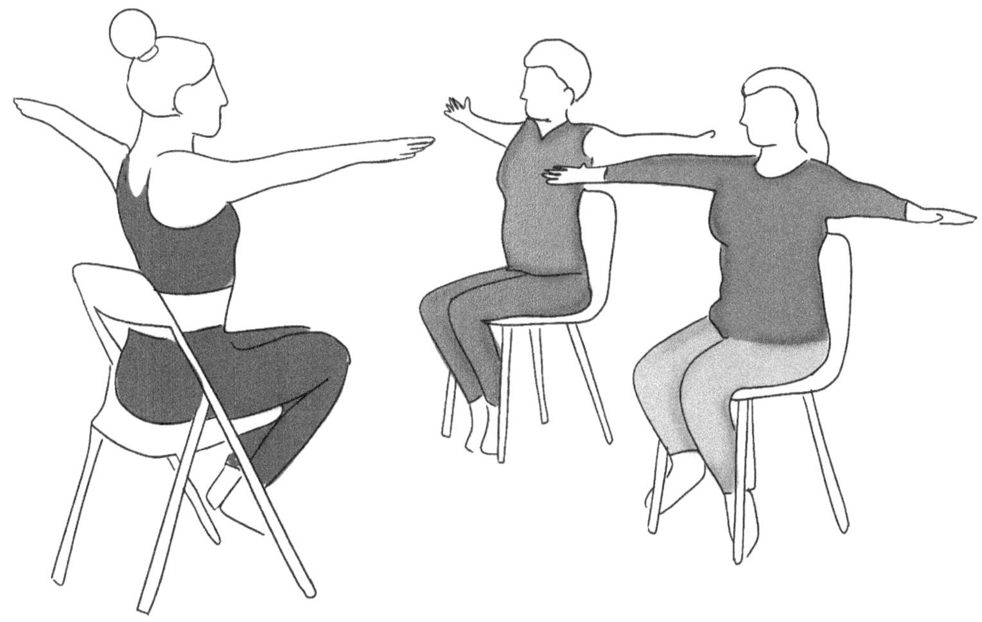

Chair yoga-assisted marching is a seated exercise that combines the benefits of chair yoga and marching movements. It is a low-impact activity suitable for individuals with limited mobility or those who may find standing exercises challenging.

To perform a chair yoga-assisted march:

✓ Sit comfortably on a sturdy chair with your feet flat on the floor, hip-width apart, and your hands resting on your thighs.
✓ Also, activate your core muscles and keep an upright posture throughout the exercise.
✓ Lift one foot slightly off the floor, then lower it back down.
✓ Do the same movement with the other foot, creating a marching motion while seated.
✓ As you lift each foot, you can also swing your opposite arm forward, similar to walking.
✓ Keep on alternating between your right and left foot, maintaining a steady and controlled pace.
✓ Breathe naturally and focus on the movements to stay mindful and engaged during the exercise.

Chair yoga-assisted march helps improve circulation, strengthen leg muscles, and promote flexibility while providing the benefits of a mild cardiovascular workout.

Seated Kick and Punch

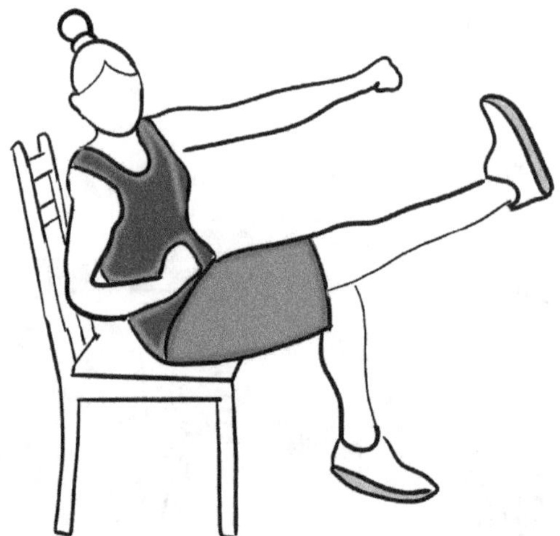

Seated kick and punch is a seated exercise routine that involves performing kicking and punching movements while remaining seated on a chair. It's a modified form of cardio workout that can be done by individuals who have limited mobility or prefer a low-impact exercise option.

To perform seated kicks and punches:

Sit comfortably on a sturdy chair with your back straight and yor feet flat on the floor.

For kicking

Lift one leg off the ground and extend it straight out in front of you, as if you are kicking forward. Bring the leg back down to the starting position. Repeat with the other leg.

For punching

Make fists with your hands and put them at chest level. Extend one arm straight out in front of you as if you are punching forward. Bring the arm back to the first position. Do the same with the other arm.

Other tips:

✓ Continue alternating between the kicking and punching movements, creating a fluid motion.
✓ Maintain your movements well controlled and activate your core for stability.
✓ Breathe steadily throughout the exercise.

Seated kicks and punches help improve cardiovascular endurance, strengthen upper and lower body muscles, and enhance coordination and balance.

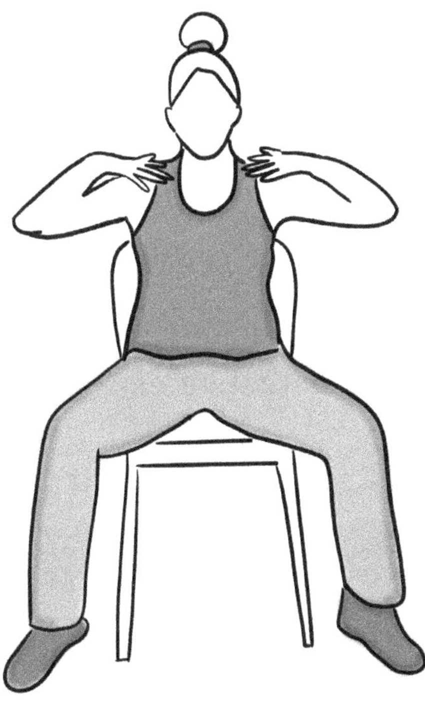

Chair yoga cardio Press and Open exercises are two movements that can be combined to create a dynamic seated workout, providing a cardiovascular challenge while promoting flexibility and upper body strength. These exercises are suitable for individuals who prefer or require a seated exercise option.

Chair Yoga Cardio Press:

✓ As a first thing, you should sit upright on a chair with your feet flat on the ground and your hands along your thighs.
✓ Take a deep breath in and raise your arms out to the sides, placing them up to shoulder level.
✓ Exhale and press your palms in front of your chest, as if you are in a prayer position.
✓ Inhale one more time and open your arms wide, stretching them out to the sides and back to shoulder level.
✓ Exhale and return to the starting position with your hands resting on your thighs.
✓ Do this sequence again for a set number of repetitions or as long as you feel comfortable.

Chair Yoga Cardio Open:

✓ Begin in the same seated position as before, with your feet flat on the floor and your hands resting on your thighs.
✓ Inhale in a deep way and reach your arms straight out in front of you, parallel to the floor.
✓ Exhale and open your arms wide to the sides, stretching them out as far as you comfortably can.
✓ Inhale one more time and put your arms back in front, parallel to the floor.
✓ Exhale and return your arms to the starting position with your hands resting on your thighs.
✓ Repeat this sequence for a set number of repetitions or as long as you feel comfortable.

Both exercises can be performed in a continuous flow, moving from Chair Yoga Cardio Press to Chair Yoga Cardio Open and back again, creating a rhythmic and dynamic workout routine. Remember to maintain proper posture, engage your core, and breathe steadily throughout the exercises.

Alternate Kick

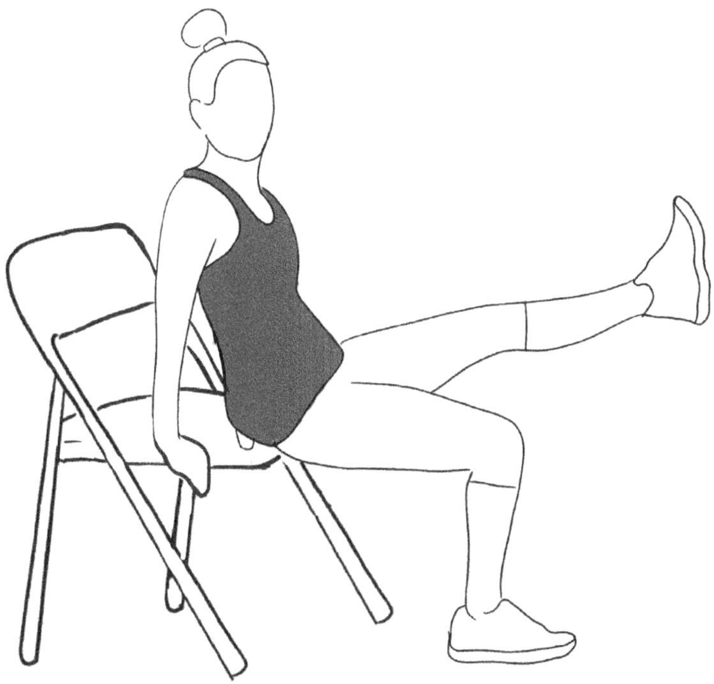

Chair yoga alternate kick exercises are seated movements that involve lifting and extending one leg at a time while remaining seated on a chair. These exercises help promote leg strength, flexibility, and balance, making them suitable for individuals with limited mobility or those who prefer a seated workout.

Chair yoga alternate kick exercises are a gentle way to activate and strengthen the leg muscles while providing a mild cardio workout.

Let's see how to perform chair yoga alternate kick exercises:

✓ Sit comfortably on a sturdy chair with your back straight and your feet flat on the ground.
✓ Put your hands on the sides of the chair or on your thighs for support.
✓ Lift one foot off the floor, keeping your knee bent at a 90-degree angle.
✓ Extend your leg forward, kicking it out in front of you as much as your flexibility allows.
✓ Hold the extended position briefly, engaging your quadriceps (front thigh muscles).
✓ Put your foot back down on the floor.
✓ Do the same movement with the other leg, alternating between left and right.
✓ Aim for a smooth and controlled motion, maintaining stability and balance throughout.
✓ Continue alternating leg kicks for a set number of repetitions or as long as you feel comfortable.
✓ Do not forget to breathe steadily and pay attention to maintaining proper form during the exercise.

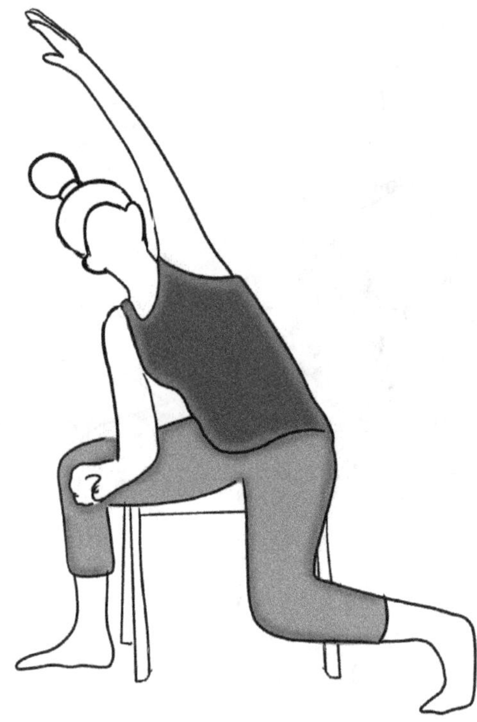

Chair yoga step-out exercises are a set of movements designed to engage the lower body muscles and promote flexibility while remaining seated on a chair. These exercises are particularly helpful for individuals with limited mobility or those seeking a gentle seated workout.

We are going to give you a full list of how to perform chair yoga step-out exercises:

✓ Sit comfortably on a sturdy chair with your feet flat on the floor and your hands resting on your thighs or on the sides of the chair for support.
✓ Begin with your feet together and your knees facing forward.
✓ Step your right foot out to the side, keeping your foot flat on the floor.
✓ Put your right foot again in the primary position beside your left foot.
✓ Now, step your left foot out to the side, again keeping it flat on the floor.
✓ Return your left foot to the beginning position beside your right foot.
✓ Continue this stepping motion, alternating between your right and left foot, like a gentle side-to-side movement.
✓ As you step out, keep your movements slow and controlled, engaging your leg muscles.
✓ Breathe steadily and keep an upright posture during the exercise's execution.
✓ You can adjust the pace and range of motion based on your comfort level and mobility.

Chair yoga step-out exercises help promote circulation, improve range of motion in the hips, and provide a subtle workout for the leg muscles.

On the other side, Chair yoga knee tap exercises are seated movements that focus on engaging the core muscles and promoting flexibility in the hips and knees.

So, we want you to understand how to perform chair yoga knee tap exercises:

✓ Sit comfortably on a sturdy chair with your back straight and your feet flat on the floor.
✓ Put your hands on the sides of the chair or on your thighs for support.
✓ Begin by lifting your right foot off the floor and bringing your knee towards your chest.
✓ Gently tap your right knee with your right hand, reaching towards your knee as much as you comfortably can.
✓ Come back again with your right foot placed on the floor.
✓ Repeat the same movement on the left side, lifting your left foot, tapping your left knee with your left hand, and then lowering your left foot back to the floor.
✓ Continue alternating between right and left knee taps for a set number of repetitions or as long as you feel comfortable.
✓ Remember to breathe steadily and engage your core muscles during the movement.

Chair yoga knee tap exercises help strengthen the core and hip flexor muscles while also enhancing balance and coordination.

Final thoughts about chair yoga as cardio-focused exercises for weight loss

Chair yoga as a cardio-focused exercise can be a beneficial addition to a weight loss journey, especially for individuals with limited mobility or those looking for low-impact options. While chair yoga may not be as intense as traditional high-impact cardio exercises, it can still contribute to weight loss and overall well-being in several ways:

✓ Cardiovascular Benefits: Chair yoga exercises with a cardio focus can elevate the heart rate, leading to improved cardiovascular health. Engaging in regular cardio activities, even in a seated position, can aid in burning calories and promoting weight loss.
✓ Muscle Engagement: Chair yoga involves various movements that engage different muscle groups, such as the core, legs, and arms. Strengthening these muscles can lead to increased metabolism and calorie burning, supporting weight loss efforts.
✓ Mind-Body Connection: Chair yoga emphasizes mindfulness and breath control, which can help reduce stress and emotional eating. By fostering a stronger mind-body connection, individuals may become more attuned to their bodies' needs and make healthier choices.
✓ Sustainable Exercise: Chair yoga is gentle on the joints and accessible to people of various fitness levels and ages. It offers a low-impact option that can be sustained over time, promoting consistency in workouts, which is key for weight loss success.
✓ Overall Well-being: consistent chair yoga practice can bring to a more flexibility, balance, and posture, reducing the risk of injury when you are practicing other physical activities. Feeling better physically and emotionally may also motivate individuals to engage in healthier lifestyle choices.

However, it's essential to remember that weight loss primarily ups to the balance between calorie intake and expenditure. Incorporating chair yoga as part of an overall weight loss plan, along with a healthy diet and other physical activities, can lead to more effective and sustainable results.

28-DAY CHALLENGE: LIFESTYLE AND NUTRITIONAL TIPS FOR WEIGHT LOSS

And here we are at the final part of this guide on chair yoga. We have covered everything related to the exercises, how to perform them, and which ones to focus on to obtain weight loss while at the same time increasing muscle tone. In this final part, however, we will talk about nutrition. We are also offering you a complete 28-day challenge where there is a perfect combination of chair yoga and proper nutrition.

Chair yoga and a better lifestyle

Chair yoga, as we have seen more and more times, that is a great way to incorporate physical activity into a sedentary lifestyle. It allows you to do yoga poses and stretches while seated on a chair, making it accessible to people with mobility or balance issues. Coupled with a balanced diet and consistent exercise, it can lead to a better and healthier lifestyle.

Embrace chair yoga in your daily routine

Incorporating chair yoga into your daily routine can bring numerous benefits to your physical and mental well-being. Let's see, one by one, some steps to embrace chair yoga in your daily life:

1. Set a Schedule: Dedicate a specific time each day for your chair yoga practice. Consistency is key to reaping the benefits.
2. Create a Space: Set up a comfortable and quiet area where you can practice chair yoga without distractions.
3. Start Slowly: If you're new to chair yoga, begin with simple poses and gradually increase the difficulty level as you become more comfortable.
4. Follow Guided Sessions: Use online resources or mobile apps that offer guided chair

yoga sessions. This can be an optimal idea for keeping you motivated and learning new poses.

5. Listen to Your Body: Never push yourself beyond your limits and modify poses if needed.
6. Breathe Mindfully: Be committed to your breath during the practice to improve relaxation and reduce stress.
7. Set Goals: state realistic goals for your chair yoga practice, such as improving flexibility or reducing tension.
8. Stay Positive: Embrace a positive mindset and celebrate your progress, no matter how little it may be.

By adding chair yoga to your daily routine, you can enjoy its physical and mental benefits and move towards a healthier lifestyle. We want you to always keep in mind that consistency and patience are keys to making positive changes in your well-being.

How to have the right mentality for weight loss

Having the right mentality for weight loss is essential for achieving your goals and maintaining a healthy lifestyle. For this purpose, we want to show you some useful tips to cultivate a positive mindset:

- ✓ Again, and always: Establish realistic goals. Set achievable and precise weight loss goals. Unrealistic expectations can lead to frustration and demotivation.
- ✓ Focus on Health, Not Just Appearance: Shift your focus from solely appearance-based goals to improving your overall health and well-being.
- ✓ Practice Self-Compassion: Be kind to yourself throughout the weight loss journey. Avoid self-criticism and be happy with your progress, every time!
- ✓ Stay Patient: Weight loss may require lots of time and so many efforts, so it's essential to remain patient during this path.
- ✓ Adopt a Balanced Diet: Focus on a balanced and nutritious diet instead of crash diets.
- ✓ Incorporate Regular Exercise: Find physical activities you enjoy, as it can make the weight loss journey more enjoyable and sustainable.
- ✓ Manage Stress: Develop healthy coping mechanisms for stress, as emotional eating can hinder weight loss progress.
- ✓ Surround Yourself with Supportive People: Seek support from friends, family, or a weight loss community to stay motivated and accountable.
- ✓ Practice Mindful Eating: Savor your meals and enjoy the eating experience.
- ✓ Focus on Non-Scale Victories: Acknowledge and celebrate other achievements beyond the number on the scale, such as improved energy levels or better sleep.
- ✓ Learn from Setbacks: If you face challenges or setbacks, you should visualize them as chances to learn and grow rather than as failures.

And, as final tips, it's necessary to take into consideration that weight loss is not just about physical changes but also about creating healthy habits and a positive relationship with your body. Having a healthy mentality and mindset will contribute to long-term success and a happier, healthier life.

Chair yoga weight loss tips

While, as we have seen previously in this book, chair yoga may not cause as much calorie consumption as high-intensity exercises do, it can still be a valuable component of a weight loss journey. And don't forget that, while chair yoga can be beneficial for weight loss, it's essential to combine it with a balanced diet and a comprehensive approach to fitness to achieve the best results. Always prioritize your safety and well-being, and make any necessary adjustments to your routine based on your individual circumstances.

But we think it's right to show you, at this point in the guide, some chair yoga tips to aid in weight loss:

- ✓ Consistency: Incorporate chair yoga into your daily routine or at least several times a week to make it a regular part of your physical activity.
- ✓ Increase Intensity: Look for chair yoga sequences that incorporate more dynamic movements and challenging poses to elevate your heart rate and increase calorie burn.
- ✓ Combine with Other Activities: Use chair yoga as a complement to other forms of exercise, such as walking or strength training, to create a well-rounded fitness routine.
- ✓ Mindful Eating: Combine your chair yoga practice with mindful eating habits to develop a better understanding of your hunger cues and avoid overeating.
- ✓ Focus on Core Engagement: During chair yoga poses, engage your core muscles to strengthen your abdominal area and improve posture.
- ✓ Practice Deep Breathing: Breathing exercises in chair yoga can help reduce stress, which may lead to less emotional eating.
- ✓ Gradual Progression: As you become more comfortable with chair yoga, challenge yourself with more advanced poses or longer sequences to boost your physical activity level.
- ✓ Seek Variety: Explore different chair yoga routines to keep your practice enjoyable and engaging.
- ✓ Monitor Progress: Keep track of your chair yoga sessions and observe any changes in your flexibility, strength, or overall well-being.
- ✓ Consult a Professional: If you have specific weight loss goals, consider consulting with a healthcare professional or a certified yoga instructor who can tailor a chair yoga program to your needs.

General nutritional tips for weight loss

To give you a helping hand, we have collected all the most useful and general nutritional tips for weight loss. Among these, all you should take into account are:

- ✓ Lead the way to a Calorie Deficit: To lose weight, it's necessary to consume fewer calories than your body burns. Focus on obtaining a calorie deficit thanks to the combination of diet and exercise.
- ✓ Eat Balanced Meals like fruits, vegetables, whole grains, lean proteins, and healthy fats to ensure you're getting essential nutrients.

✓ Control Portion Sizes: Always pay more attention to portion sizes and stay away from overeating.

✓ Limit Added Sugars and Processed Foods: Reduce your intake of sugary beverages, sweets, and highly processed foods, as they can contribute to weight gain.

✓ Stay Hydrated: Drink a lot of water; it's the key. Sometimes, in fact, thirst can be thought of as hunger, but in reality it's not.

✓ Prioritize Protein: Including protein in your meals can help you feel fuller for longer and maintain muscle mass during weight loss.

✓ Choose Healthy Fats: So, look for sources of healthy fats like avocados, nuts, seeds, and olive oil, which can help keep you satisfied.

✓ Eat Mindfully: As we have said above, be focused on what you eat and savor each bite.

✓ Plan Ahead: Set your meals and snacks beforehand to avoid impulsive food choices, especially when you're hungry.

✓ Don't Skip Meals: never do it, because this mistake can lead to overeating later in the day. Aim for regular, balanced meals and incorporate healthy snacks if needed.

✓ Be Patient and avoid quick diets or huge restrictions, as they are often not maintainable in the long term.

✓ Get Adequate Sleep: Lack of sleep can interfere with weight loss efforts. Try to obtain a quality sleep for about 7-9 hours each night.

✓ Never forget that it's essential to find a nutritional approach that fits your individual needs and preferences. And this can lead you to ask a registered dietitian or healthcare professional to give you some personalized guidance and support on your weight loss journey.

28-day challenges: chair yoga and nutritional tips

A 28-day challenge combining chair yoga and nutritional tips can be a great way to kickstart your journey towards a healthier lifestyle. Here's a plan to get you started:

Week 1 - Getting into the Routine:

1. Chair Yoga: Start with a gentle 15-minute chair yoga session every morning. Focus on basic stretches and poses to ease into the practice.
2. Nutritional Tips: the first thing you can do is tracking your daily food intake with the aid of a mobile app or a journal. Pay attention to portion sizes and aim for balanced meals with fruits, vegetables, lean proteins, and whole grains.

Week 2 - Building Momentum:

✓ Chair Yoga: Increase the duration of your chair yoga sessions to 20-25 minutes. Add more dynamic exercises and stretches to challenge yourself.

✓ Nutritional Tips: Continue tracking your meals and start decreasing your amount of added sugars and processed foods. Look for healthier snacks such us fruits, nuts, or yogurt.

Week 3 - Deepening the Practice:

✓ Chair Yoga: Try more intermediate chair yoga poses and sequences, focusing on strengthening your core and improving flexibility.
✓ Nutritional Tips: Experiment with new healthy recipes and cooking methods. Add more plant-based meals into your daily nutrition, like salads and vegetable stir-fries.

Week 4 - Embracing the Challenge:

✓ Chair Yoga: By now, you should feel more comfortable with chair yoga. Try longer sessions, up to 30 minutes, and challenge yourself with advanced poses if you feel ready.
✓ Nutritional Tips: Focus on mindful eating during this week. Pay attention to hunger and fullness cues, and practice eating slowly and savoring your meals.

Throughout the 28-day challenge

Let's see other tips to follow during this challenge period:

✓ Hydration: Drink huge amount of this essential element throughout the day to keep your body hydrated and give some help to your body's functions.
✓ Self-Reflection: Take time each day to reflect on your progress, both in chair yoga and your dietary choices.
✓ Rest Days: Incorporate rest days for your body to recover and rejuvenate. On these days, you can still practice gentle chair yoga or take a short walk.
✓ Accountability: Share your challenge with a friend or join an online community where you can find support, motivation, and share experiences.
✓ Never forget that the key to success is consistency and making gradual changes. Enjoy the process and celebrate every step towards a healthier and happier you!

Final thoughts on a challenge that combines chair yoga and weight loss

Combining chair yoga with weight loss in a challenge is a fantastic way to promote holistic well-being. Chair yoga offers a gentle yet effective form of exercise accessible to people of various fitness levels, including those with limited mobility. Pairing chair yoga with weight loss goals allows for a balanced approach to overall health. While chair yoga may not burn as many calories as high-intensity exercises, it contributes to physical and mental well-being, making it easier to stay consistent with other aspects of weight loss, such as a healthy diet.

A successful chair yoga and weight loss challenge should focus on gradual progress, mindful eating, and self-compassion. Keep always in mind that weight loss is a journey, and positive changes take time. Celebrate each small victory and learn from setbacks without being too hard on yourself.

The challenge offers an opportunity to discover the joy of movement, mindfulness, and self-care. By combining chair yoga with nutritional tips, you'll create a sustainable lifestyle that goes beyond mere weight loss and leads to improved overall health, increased self-awareness, and a deeper connection with your body.

Embrace the challenge with an open mind, dedication, and a willingness to grow. Enjoy the path, and may it bring you closer to a healthier, happier, and more balanced life.

CONCLUSIONS

In this book we have addressed with care and dedication a very important topic that could help most of us in our daily lives: chair yoga. Let's see together what main topics we discussed.

For doing this, we want to show you a final summary of some main chair yoga topics:

- ✓ Chair Yoga Poses: Explore a variety of yoga poses that can be modified for seated practice. These include gentle stretches, twists, forward bends, and balance exercises that can be done while sitting on a chair.
- ✓ Mindfulness and Meditation: Discover techniques to cultivate mindfulness and meditation in a seated position, fostering mental clarity and emotional well-being.
- ✓ Flexibility and Mobility: Focus on improving flexibility, range of motion, and joint health through chair yoga movements.
- ✓ Strength and Balance: Engage in poses and exercises that help build strength and enhance balance, benefiting overall stability and posture.
- ✓ Stress Reduction: Understand how chair yoga can be an effective tool for managing stress, promoting relaxation, and calming the mind.
- ✓ Adaptations for Special Populations: Learn about chair yoga modifications suitable for seniors, individuals with limited mobility, or those recovering from injuries.
- ✓ Chair Yoga Routines: Discover pre-designed chair yoga sequences to follow, offering a structured and balanced practice.
- ✓ Integrating Chair Yoga into Daily Life: Explore ways to incorporate chair yoga into daily routines, including at work, during travel, or at home.
- ✓ Benefits of Chair Yoga: Understand the physical, mental, and emotional benefits of practicing chair yoga regularly.

We have divided our book into these main chair yoga topics, and this for allow you to cultivate a comprehensive understanding of this accessible and beneficial practice. In this conclusion we want you to remind to approach chair yoga with an open mind, listen to your body's cues, and consult a qualified instructor or healthcare professional if needed.

Chair yoga is an incredibly useful and versatile practice that brings numerous benefits to people from all walks of life. Its adaptability makes it accessible for individuals with limited mobility, seniors, office workers, and anyone looking for a gentle yet effective form of exercise and relaxation. By incorporating chair yoga into your daily routine, you can experience improved flexibility, strength, and balance while reducing stress and promoting mindfulness. Its ease and convenience make it a practical option for incorporating yoga into busy schedules or for those who may find traditional yoga challenging. Embracing chair yoga opens the door to a healthier and more mindful lifestyle, enhancing overall well-being and fostering a deeper connection with oneself. So, regardless of age or physical ability, chair yoga presents a valuable opportunity to nurture both body and mind, making it a practice worth exploring and embracing.

We have also understood that, while chair yoga offers numerous health benefits, it's essential to have realistic expectations regarding its role in weight loss. Chair yoga can be a valuable addition to a weight loss journey, as it promotes flexibility, strength, and mindful awareness of the body's needs. It can bring to a better overall well-being, which may, even in a softer way, support weight loss efforts.

However, for significant weight loss, a comprehensive approach that includes a balanced diet, regular physical activity, and lifestyle changes is crucial. Chair yoga can complement these efforts by increasing physical activity levels and fostering a positive mindset.

Remember, weight loss success is a result of multiple factors working together, and chair yoga can be a helpful tool in your wellness toolkit.

Having said this, if you're looking to learn more about chair yoga and deepen your understanding, here are some additional sources you can explore:

1. Books: Look for books dedicated to chair yoga, written by experienced yoga instructors or experts in the field. They often provide detailed explanations, illustrations, and practice sequences. Check online bookstores or local libraries for titles like "Chair Yoga: Sit, Stretch, and Strengthen Your Way to a Happier, Healthier You" by Kristin McGee or "Chair Yoga: Seated Exercises for Health and Wellbeing" by Edeltraud Rohnfeld.
2. Online Courses: Various online platforms offer chair yoga courses taught by certified instructors. These courses may include video lessons, practice sessions, and in-depth explanations of poses and techniques. Websites like Udemy, Coursera, or Yoga International might have relevant courses to explore.
3. YouTube: YouTube is a vast resource for free chair yoga videos. Many skilled yoga instructors offer instructional sessions suitable for all levels. Search for "chair yoga" or specific instructors' channels to find valuable content.
4. Online Yoga Communities: Join online forums, Facebook groups, or other social media platforms that are all about yoga. These communities often share insights, experiences, and resources related to chair yoga.
5. Local Yoga Studios and Senior Centers: Check if any yoga studios or senior centers in your area offer chair yoga classes. Attending in-person sessions can provide hands-on guidance and personalized instruction.
6. Mobile Apps: Some mobile apps cater specifically to chair yoga and offer guided sessions, practice routines, and tips for beginners. Look for apps like "Chair Yoga" or "Yoga for Seniors."
7. Research Articles: To explore the scientific benefits of chair yoga, you can search for

research articles on platforms like PubMed or Google Scholar. These studies delve into the impacts of chair yoga on various aspects of health and well-being.

In conclusion, chair yoga offers a wonderful and accessible way for people of all ages and abilities to obtain the same benefits of yoga. By incorporating gentle stretches, breathwork, and mindfulness exercises while seated, it promotes flexibility, relaxation, and improved overall well-being. Whether you're a beginner, have limited mobility, or simply looking for a convenient practice, chair yoga can be a valuable addition to your daily routine. So, embrace the benefits of this adaptable practice and embark on a journey of enhanced physical and mental health through the ease and comfort of your chair. Namaste!

✷ DEAR VALUED READER,

Thank you for choosing "Chair Yoga for Seniors Over 60"
to embark on your wellness journey!

Your feedback is incredibly valuable to me!

★ LEAVE A REVIEW:

Your thoughts mean the world to me. If you liked the
book, please take a moment to share your experience
by leaving a review. Your words inspire and guide me
in creating content that truly makes a difference.

👇 SCAN HERE TO LEAVE YOUR REVIEW* 👇

As a token of gratitude, I'm thrilled to offer you a fantastic bonus:

✨ COMPLIMENTARY INTERACTIVE PROGRESS TRACKER ✨

📊 TRACK YOUR WEIGHT LOSS, MEASURE YOUR PROGRESS, AND CELEBRATE EACH WELLNESS MILESTONE WITH OUR INTERACTIVE PDF TRACKER.

🎁 DOWNLOAD YOUR FREE BONUS NOW!

Scan the QR Code Below

* Optional